The Anti-Inflammatory Diet cookbook for beginners:

The best beginner's guide, nearly 100 Easy Recipes to Heal the Immune System and Restore Overall Health.

|2021 Edition|

© Copyright 2021 by Diet Academy

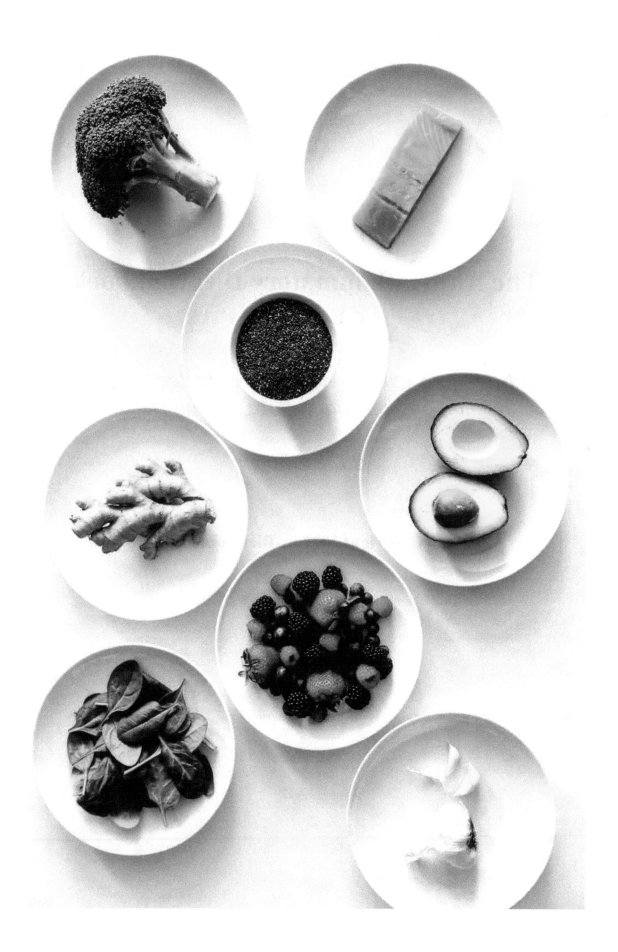

Table of Contents

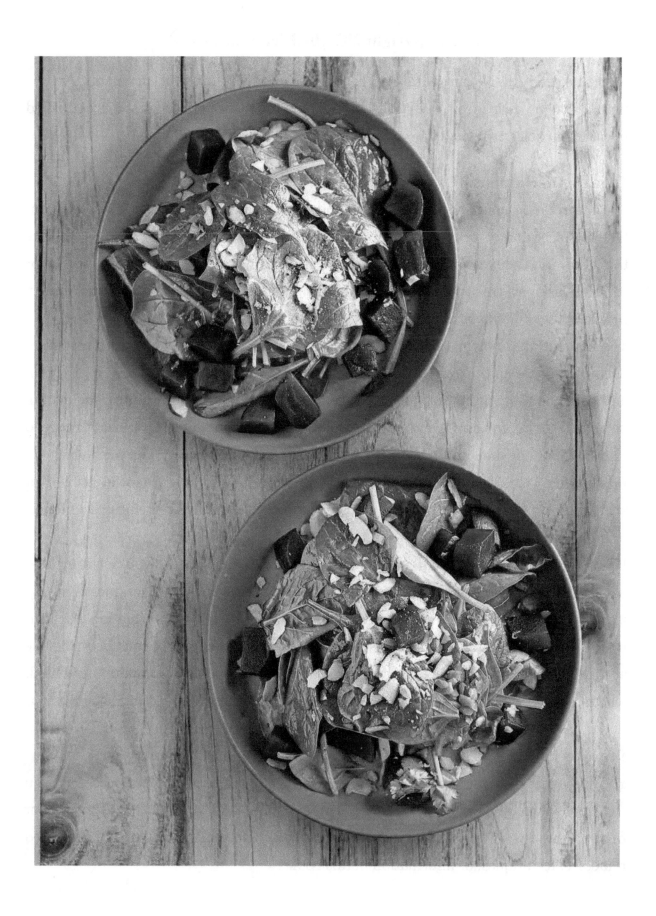

Introduction

The anti-inflammatory diet is not merely a meal plan to maintain within a limited duration; additionally, it is not solely weight loss program as well.

Nevertheless, you can indeed lose weight by practicing it. Instead, the diet is a systematic way of choosing the right foods and preparing anti-inflammatory meals.

It derives its food selection and cooking processes on the scientific and medical knowledge of how your food intakes can help your body to attain and maintain optimum wellness. This natural dieting greatly influences the beneficial goals of inflammation.

The regimen provides you with a steady supply of energy, mainly sourced from the sufficient macronutrient consumptions. These intakes include dietary fibers and essential fatty acids. You will also have your ample share of vitamins and minerals from the micronutrient intakes.

Likewise, you can benefit more with the diet's protective phytonutrients. These are healthy and nourishing substances commonly derived from plants such as lycopene, lutein, and carotene.

People suffering from inflammatory diseases can reduce their inflammation and its side effects. They only need to radically change their diets. They can enhance the effect of taking prescribed medications with a proper nutrition program (anti-inflammatory diet).

Logically, if you intend to reduce inflammation, then consume less of the inflammatory foods.

Instead, eat more and more of the anti-inflammatory foods.

Your regimen must provide for a healthy balance of macronutrients—fats, proteins, and carbohydrates—at each meal. Ensure also to meet your body's daily requirements for fibers, water, vitamins, and minerals.

Base your anti-inflammatory diet on nutrient-rich and whole foods containing antioxidants.

These substances ably help to protect your cells from the destructive effects of oxidation.

In essence, antioxidants function by reducing the levels of free radicals. These are incredibly reactive compounds, which damage fats and proteins.

Free radicals also accelerate the progression of cardiovascular diseases, rheumatoid arthritis, cancer, radiation sickness, atherosclerosis, age-related illnesses, and many other health issues. Hence, avoid processed products, which are often dense with free radicals.

Generally, the natural design and function of the highly reactive molecules of free radicals are to assist metabolism. This biological process involves breaking down food compounds into smaller particles and disposing the absorbed nutrients into the blood to create energy for your body.

However, when you are unable to reduce or purge any intense reactions of these harmful free radicals, they can ultimately lead to inflammatory issues. You can only hold them in check through ingesting prescribed foods from the regimen.

Various Versions & Variations of The Dietary Discipline: Replacement Regimens

The anti-inflammatory diet is a natural and nutritional regimen. As such, it encompasses most dietary plans.

The diet is relative to a wide range of recommended traditional and modern nutritional regimen.

Its breadths and depths reflect the recommended food compositions.

The food elements include lots of fruits and vegetables, plant-based proteins (i.e., nuts and legumes), and fresh, organically grown herbs and spices. Whole grains and fatty fish are also among the regular staples.

If you were to account the macronutrient values, then the regimen inherently has limited calories (energy content of food), proteins, and saturated fats (solid fats). However, it is significantly rich in fibers or plant carbohydrates and trans-unsaturated fats (essential fatty acids).

Incidentally, these typical foods also form part of the core of food elements of several dietary disciplines. Three of these popular diets are the Mediterranean Diet, various types of Low-Carbohydrate Diets, and Vegan/Vegetarian Diets. Many nutritionists and dieticians consider these regimens as anti-inflammatory diets in nature.

Mediterranean Meals: The conception of the Mediterranean Diet was an inspiration of the time-honored dietary habits of people living within the Mediterranean region. The main feature of the diet is the high consumptions of olive oil, unrefined grains, legumes, fruits, and vegetables.

The regimen also includes moderate-to-high intakes of seafood and dairy products (often, yogurt and cheese). However, it restricts consuming non-fish and red meats. Its distinctive aspect emphasizes social celebrations of food with regulated intakes of wine.

Generally, it is a beneficial dietary plan rich in dietary fibers and monounsaturated fats while low in saturated fats. The Mediterranean Diet demonstrates to reduce inflammatory indicators like IL-6 and CRP.

Olive oil is the primary component of the diet that promotes good health. Studies insist that the regular consumptions of olive oil can lower mortality rates, neurodegeneration, and cardiovascular diseases. Additional studies also show that olive oil reduces the risks of cancer and several other chronic diseases.

Common Carb-Restricted Regimens: As its term implies, the dietary program emphasizes carbohydrate restriction. People often apply this typical regimen for the treatment or prevention of some chronic diseases.

These recurring health issues include high blood pressure and cardiovascular disease, gut fermentation and metabolic syndromes, and diabetes. It also reduces inflammation, especially for people who are obese.

The working principle of this diet entails limiting or replacing foods high in carbohydrates with foods that are rich in fats but moderate in proteins, as well as other foods low in carbs. The replaced food items are usually those easily digestible foods (i.e., pasta, bread, sugar, etc.), which have high glycemic indices (carb ratings that measure how quickly they raise blood sugar levels).

On one hand, these diets highly suggest consuming fatty foods with adequate protein contents. These food sources generally come from dairy, livestock, and poultry produce; nuts and seeds; and, seafood, particularly shellfish.

On the other hand, these diets recommended low-carb foods are those dark, green, and leafy vegetables. Low-carb diets also advise intakes of specific fruits, most preferably, berries.

The tolerable amounts of carb intakes vary with each specific low-carb regimen. Generally, a low-carb diet applies to meal plans that limit carb consumptions to less than 20% of one's recommended daily calorie intake.

For a steady and healthy dietary regimen, males require about 2,500 calories per day for healthy weight maintenance. Females need only to consume 2,000 calories each day. However, these figures may vary depending on age, body composition, and intensity levels of daily physical activities.

Similarly, low-carb diets may also refer to regimens that limit carb intakes to not more than the maximum recommended values. They use a rule of thumb for carb restrictions between 5% and 30% of your daily calorie intake.

The Ketogenic Diet is the chief proponent of this severe carb restriction regimen. The diet follows a regulated food consumption of 70% to 80% of calories from fats, 15% to 25% of calories from proteins, and 5% to 10% of calories from carbohydrates.

These caloric ratios fulfill the intents of inducing the body to enter into a state of ketosis. Ketosis is the occurrence of an excessive accumulation of ketones or fatty tissues in the bloodstream that the body cells use to burn for energy instead of carbohydrates.

The Atkins Diet also has a similar induction stage as the Ketogenic Diet. The only difference between these low-carb diets is the prescribed amounts of protein consumptions. The Atkins Diet proffers unlimited protein intakes along its 4-stage dietary plan.

The Paleo Diet is also a relatively low-carb regimen. It has a carb intake rating of 20% to 40% of calories from carbs.

The regimen distinctively summons the analogy of the eating patterns of our ancient ancestors who were initially hunter-gatherers. Thus, the diet mainly focuses on plant and animal foods low in carbs. Studies show that wild and organically grown plants contain fewer carbs and abundant in fiber compared to modern plant crops.

Vegan | Vegetarian Versions: Vegan and Vegetarian Diets carry the same wellness intent: to reduce inflammation. Engaging with the anti-inflammatory diet is like indulging with vegan protein sources or fatty fish instead of meat.

The principal staples of both Vegan and Vegetarian Diets are plant-based foods rich in vitamin K. These are mostly dark, green, and leafy veggies like broccoli, kale, and spinach. These leafy greens have long been heralded to help restrain inflammation.

Fresh fruits (i.e., blackberries, raspberries, etc.) are also essential food items of these plant-based regimens. The pigment that produces the specific colors for these fruits is a vital element in battling inflammation.

These versions and variations of the diet have already gained a foothold and a broader acceptance in today's society. Practitioners use them either as strategies to maintain good health or as medical nutrition therapies to manage their health issues. Nonetheless, most people commit themselves actively to these diets to seek protection against inflammatory conditions.

Summing it up, numerous studies have validated the countless health benefits of each of these regimens. For one, experts confirmed that vegetarians had increased levels of plasma amino acid (general health indicators associated with lower risks of heart disease and inflammation). In contrast, a recent study affirmed that consuming animal products increased the chances of acquiring chronic inflammation.

Chapter 1: Principles of the Anti-Inflammatory Diet

Benefits of the Anti-Inflammatory Diet

Naturopaths, dietitians, nutritionists, and physicians are always inclined to prescribe the anti-inflammatory regimen. In all likelihood, they will endorse it as a complementary therapy for several health conditions aggravated by chronic inflammation.

Since it is a widely regarded healthy diet, it helps to lessen your chances of acquiring other health problems. That is, even if the regimen does not help with your current conditions.

The principal benefit of an anti-inflammatory diet is the reduction of inflammatory indicators in the blood. Foremost, it enhances blood sugar, triglyceride, and cholesterol levels.

The dietary regimen also boosts energy while improving your overall health and moods. In conclusion, strictly following an anti-inflammatory regimen and lifestyle, together with regular physical exercise and adequate sleep, can drastically reduce your risks of incurring many diseases, to wit:

- *Active Hepatitis*
- *Alzheimer's disease*
- *Asthma*
- *Cancer, particularly Colorectal Cancer*
- *Chronic Sinusitis | Ulcerative Colitis*
- *Colitis*
- *Crohn's Disease*
- *Diabetes*
- *Eosinophilic Esophagitis*
- *Hashimoto's Disease*

- *Heart Diseases*
- *Inflammatory Bowel Syndromes (IBS)*
- *Lupus*
- *Metabolic Syndrome*
- *Obesity*
- *Peptic Ulcer*
- *Periodontitis*
- *Psoriasis*
- *Rheumatoid Arthritis*
- *Tuberculosis*

Foods to Eat and to Avoid

The anti-inflammatory diet can be restricted for specific types of foods. This is to ensure that you don't introduce things that might trigger inflammatory responses to your body. Although there are some types of foods that you should avoid with this particular diet, there is still a plethora of food groups that you are allowed to enjoy while following this diet.

Food groups	Anti-inflammation all-stars	Foods to avoid
Beans and legumes	*Black-eyed peas, red beans, pinto beans, lentils, chickpeas, and black beans*	*NA*
Fruits	*Blueberries, blackberries, raspberries, strawberries, dark red grapes, cherries, coconut, avocado, and citrus fruits*	*NA*
Allium vegetables	*Onion, garlic, chives, shallots, leeks, green onions*	*NA*
Vegetables	*Cauliflower, broccoli, and cabbage. Also, dark leafy greens like mustard greens, collard greens, kale, lettuce, and spinach. Mushrooms, squash*	*NA*
Nightshade vegetables	*Tomatoes, bell peppers, eggplants, and potatoes*	*There is no scientific evidence that shows the nightshade group of vegetables have inflammatory properties. In fact, they are a nutritional powerhouse. Thus, if an individual is sensitive to nightshade food, then it is prudent to remove it from your diet.*

Herbs and spices	*Thyme, rosemary, cinnamon, basil, garlic, ginger, turmeric, chili peppers, paprika,*	*NA*
Animal and fish products	*Oily fish like herring, salmon, tuna, mackerel, and sardines. Lean meat*	*Avoid processed meats like sausages as they contain nitrites – a form of preservative that does little good to the body.* *Red meat like burgers and steaks*
Recommended fats	*Fats from coconut, avocado, olive oils.* *Fats from nuts like almonds, pine nuts, pistachios, and walnuts. Cocoa and chocolates*	*Fats found in fried foods; vegetable oil and soybean oil, margarine, shortening, and lard.* *Fats found in whole milk, butter—consider using low-fat dairy.* *Food laden with trans-fat such as processed foods should be avoided completely.*
Recommended drinks	*Green tea* *Red wine in moderation*	*Sugary drinks* *Excessive alcohol*
Carbohydrates	*Whole grains like unrefined grains, whole wheat bread, brown rice, oatmeal.*	*Refined carbs like white bread and pastries.* *French fries* *Artificial sugar should also be avoided.*

The Science Behind the Anti-Inflammatory Diet

When your body needs to respond to an injury, it tends to mobilize an army of specialized cells to fend of the invading organism and toxins.

Once that has happened, another group of cells tend to signal to the body and let it know the fighter cells have accomplished their task and the body is allowed to stop the production of preparatory and fighter cells.

These results a sort of cleanup that clears up the leftover fighter cells from the battlefield and repairs any damage.

Simply put, there are two steps to this response:

- Pro-Inflammatory

- Anti-Inflammatory

Each cell involved in the pro stage builds on the work of the previous cells and helps to make the immune reaction stronger for any upcoming attack.

During the pro period, symptoms such as redness, swelling, itching are common.

The anti-inflammatory is the reverse of pro-inflammatory and it works to lower the effects of inflammation.

A variety of substances used to block inflammation are made from essential fatty acids, which the body isn't able to produce on its own.

These acids must be obtained through supplements or foods.

Two essential ones are Omega-3 and Omega-6.

Omega-6 tends to increase inflammation while Omega-3 helps to reduce it.

It should be noted that what I wrote above is a simplified version of the whole mechanism and there is a lot more to it.

There are various substances that play a deeper role in the whole infrastructure that allows the body to control its inflammatory mechanism.

Some of the crucial ones are:

Histamine: White blood cells near an injury tend to release a substance known as histamine. They increase the permeability of blood vessels around the wound that signals fighter cells and other substances to regulate an immune response and come to the sight of injury. Histamine also causes redness and swelling around the affected region and causes runny nose, rash, itchy eyes.

Cytokines: These are proteins that are activated by pro-inflammatory eicosanoids to signal fighter cells to gather at the injury site. They are responsible for diverting energy from the body to catalyst the healing process. Release of these substances tend to cause tiredness and decrease appetite.

C-Reactive Protein: Cytokines alongside other pro-inflammatory eicosanoids are closely involved in the activation of a substance known as C-Reactive Protein. This particular organic compound produced by the liver responds to messages that are sent out by white blood cells. The C-Reactive proteins tend to bind the site of injury and act as a sort of surveillance unit that helps to identify the invading bodies.

Leukocytes: Several types of leukocytes (also known as white blood cells) are critical to the process of neutralizing invading substances. Neutrophils, for example, are small, agile and are able to first arrive at the scene of the crime to ingest small microbes. However, large substances such as macrophages as required to tackle a large number of microbes.

There are a few more, but the gist still remains the same. When your body starts to suffer from an uncontrolled inflammation attack, the action of these and similar substances tend to get out of control, which results in extremely uncomfortable situations.

Chapter 2: Breakfast

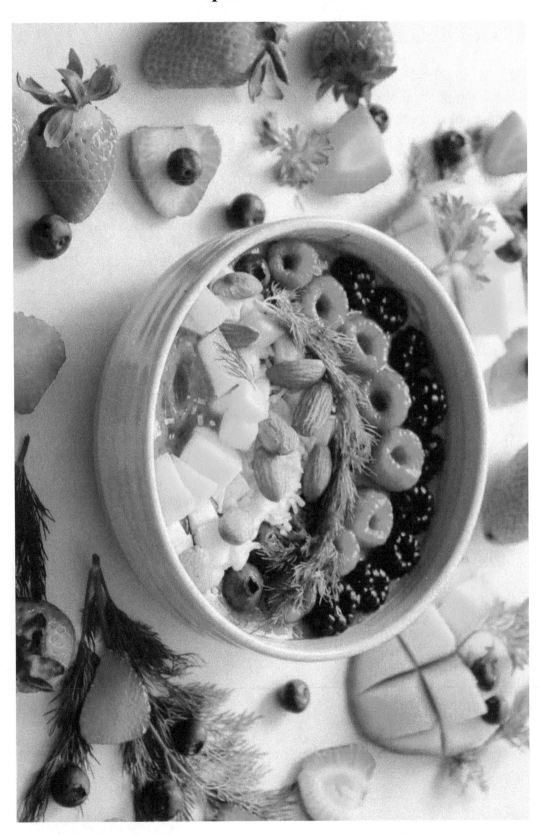

Oven-Poached Eggs

Preparation Time: 2 minutes

Cooking Time: 11 minutes

Servings: 4

Ingredients:

✓ 6 eggs, at room temperature

✓ Water

✓ Ice bath

✓ 2 cups water, chilled

✓ 2 cups of ice cubes

Directions:

Set the oven to 350°F. Put 2 cups of water into a deep roasting tin, and place it into the lowest rack of the oven.

Place one egg into each cup of cupcake/muffin tins, along with one tablespoon of water.

Carefully place muffin tins into the middle rack of the oven.

Bake eggs for 45 minutes.

Turn off the heat immediately. Take off the muffin tins from the oven and set on a cake rack to cool before extracting eggs.

Pour ice bath ingredients into a large heat-resistant bowl.

Bring the eggs into an ice bath to stop the cooking process. After 10 minutes, drain eggs well. Use as needed.

Nutrition:

✓ Calories: 357 kcal

✓ Protein: 17.14 g

✓ Fat: 24.36 g

✓ Carbohydrates: 16.19 g

Cranberry and Raisins Granola

Preparation Time: 15 minutes

Cooking Time: 20 minutes

Servings: 4

Ingredients:

- ✓ 4 cups old-fashioned rolled oats
- ✓ 1/4 cup sesame seeds
- ✓ 1 cup dried cranberries
- ✓ 1 cup golden raisins
- ✓ 1/8 teaspoon nutmeg
- ✓ 2 tablespoons olive oil
- ✓ 1/2 cup almonds, slivered
- ✓ 2 tablespoons warm water
- ✓ 1 teaspoon vanilla extract
- ✓ 1 teaspoon cinnamon
- ✓ 1/4 teaspoon of salt
- ✓ 6 tablespoons maple syrup
- ✓ 1/3 cup of honey

Directions:

In a bowl, mix the sesame seeds, nutmeg, almonds, oats, salt, and cinnamon.

In another bowl, mix the oil, water, vanilla, honey, and syrup. Gradually pour the mixture into the oats mixture. Toss to combine. Spread the mixture into a greased jelly-roll pan. Bake in the oven at 300°F for at least 55 minutes. Stir and break the clumps every 10 minutes.

Once you get it from the oven, stir the cranberries and raisins. Allow cooling. This will last for a week when stored in an airtight container and up to a month when stored in the fridge.

Nutrition:

- ✓ Calories: 698 kcal
- ✓ Protein: 21.34 g
- ✓ Fat: 20.99 g
- ✓ Carbohydrates: 148.59 g

Spicy Marble Eggs

Preparation Time: 15 minutes
Cooking Time: 2 hours
Servings: 12

Ingredients:

- ✓ 6 medium-boiled eggs, unpeeled, cooled
- ✓ For the Marinade
- ✓ 2 oolong black tea bags
- ✓ 3 Tbsp. brown sugar
- ✓ 1 thumb-sized fresh ginger, unpeeled, crushed
- ✓ 3 dried star anise, whole
- ✓ 2 dried bay leaves
- ✓ 3 Tbsp. light soy sauce
- ✓ 4 Tbsp. dark soy sauce
- ✓ 4 cups of water
- ✓ 1 dried cinnamon stick, whole
- ✓ 1 tsp. salt
- ✓ 1 tsp. dried Szechuan peppercorns

Directions:

Using the back of a metal spoon, crack eggshells in places to create a spider web effect. Do not peel. Set aside until needed.

Pour marinade into large Dutch oven set over high heat. Put lid partially on. Bring water to a rolling boil, about 5 minutes. Turn off heat.

Secure lid. Steep ingredients for 10 minutes.

Using a slotted spoon, fish out and discard solids. Cool marinade completely to room proceeding.

Place eggs into an airtight non-reactive container just small enough to snugly fit all these in.

Pour in marinade. Eggs should be completely submerged in liquid. Discard leftover marinade, if any. Line container rim with generous layers of saran wrap. Secure container lid.

Chill eggs for 24 hours before using.

Extract eggs and drain each piece well before using, but keep the rest submerged in the marinade.

Nutrition:

Calories: 75 kcal; Protein: 4.05 g; Fat: 4.36 g; Carbohydrates: 4.83 g

Nutty Oats Pudding

Preparation Time: 5 minutes

Cooking Time: 0 minutes

Servings: 3 -5

Ingredients:

- ✓ ¼ cup rolled oats
- ✓ 1 tablespoon yogurt, fat-free
- ✓ 1 ½ tablespoon natural peanut butter
- ✓ ¼ cup dry milk
- ✓ 1 teaspoon peanuts, finely chopped
- ✓ cup of water

Directions:

Using a microwaveable-safe bowl, put together peanut butter and dry milk. Whisk well. Add in water to achieve a smooth consistency. Add in oats.

Cover bowl with plastic wrap. Create a small hole for the steam to escape.

Place inside the microwave oven for 1 minute on high powder.

Continue heating, this time on medium power for 90 seconds. Let sit for 5 minutes. To serve, spoon an equal amount of cereals in a bowl top with peanuts and yogurt.

Nutrition:

- ✓ Calories: 70 kcal
- ✓ Protein: 4.25 g
- ✓ Fat: 3.83 g
- ✓ Carbohydrates: 6.78 g

Beef Breakfast Casserole

Preparation Time: 10 minutes

Cooking Time: 30 minutes

Servings: 5

Ingredients:

- ✓ 1 pound of ground beef, cooked
- ✓ 10 eggs
- ✓ cup Pico de Gallo
- ✓ 1 cup baby spinach
- ✓ ¼ cup sliced black olives Freshly ground black pepper

Directions:

Preheat oven to 350 degrees Fahrenheit. Prepare a 9" glass pie plate with non-stick spray. Whisk the eggs until frothy. Season with salt and pepper.

Layer the cooked ground beef, Pico de Gallo, and spinach in the pie plate. Slowly pour the eggs over the top.

Top with black olives.

Bake for at least 30 minutes, until firm in the middle.

Slice into 5 pieces and serve.

Nutrition:

- ✓ Calories: 479 kcal
- ✓ Protein: 43.54 g
- ✓ Fat: 30.59 g
- ✓ Carbohydrates: 4.65 g

Ham and Veggie Frittata Muffins

Preparation Time: 10 minutes

Cooking Time: 25 minutes

Servings: 12

Ingredients:

- ✓ 5 ounces thinly sliced ham
- ✓ 8 large eggs
- ✓ 4 tablespoons coconut oil
- ✓ ½ yellow onion, finely diced
- ✓ 8 oz. frozen spinach, thawed and drained
- ✓ 8 oz. mushrooms, thinly sliced
- ✓ 1 cup cherry tomatoes, halved
- ✓ cup coconut milk (canned)
- ✓ 2 tablespoons coconut flour Sea salt and pepper to taste

Directions:

Preheat oven to 375 degrees Fahrenheit.

In a medium skillet, warm the coconut oil on medium heat. Add the onion and cook until softened.

Add the mushrooms, spinach, and cherry tomatoes. Season with salt and pepper. Cook until the mushrooms have softened. About 5 minutes. Remove from heat and set aside.

In a huge bowl, beat the eggs together with the coconut milk and coconut flour. Stir in the cooled the veggie mixture.

Line each cavity of a 12 cavity muffin tin with the thinly sliced ham. Pour the egg mixture into each one and bake for 20 minutes.

Remove from oven and allow to cool for about 5 minutes before transferring to a wire rack. To maximize the benefit of a vegetable-rich diet, it's important to eat a variety of colors, and these veggie-packed frittata muffins do just that. The onion, spinach, mushrooms, and cherry tomatoes provide a wide range of vitamins and nutrients and a healthy dose of fiber.

Nutrition:

Calories: 125 kcal; Protein: 5.96 g; Fat: 9.84 g; Carbohydrates: 4.48 g

Tomato and Avocado Omelet

Preparation Time: 5 minutes

Cooking Time: 5 minutes

Servings: 1

Ingredients:

✓ 2 eggs

✓ ¼ avocado, diced

✓ 4 cherry tomatoes, halved

✓ 1 tablespoon cilantro, chopped

✓ Squeeze of lime juice

✓ Pinch of salt

Directions:

Put together the avocado, tomatoes, cilantro, lime juice, and salt in a small bowl, then mix well and set aside.

Warm a medium nonstick skillet on medium heat. Whisk the eggs until frothy and add to the pan. Move the eggs around gently with a rubber spatula until they begin to set.

Scatter the avocado mixture over half of the omelet. Remove from heat, and slide the omelet onto a plate as you fold it in half.

Serve immediately.

Nutrition:

✓ Calories: 433 kcal

✓ Protein: 25.55 g

✓ Fat: 32.75 g

✓ Carbohydrates: 10.06 g

Vegan-Friendly Banana Bread

Preparation Time: 15 minutes

Cooking Time: 40 minutes
Servings: 4-6

Ingredients:

2 ripe bananas, mashed

1/3 cup brewed coffee

3 tbsp. chia seeds

6 tbsp. water

½ cup soft vegan butter

½ cup maple syrup

2 cups flour

2 tsp. baking powder

1 tsp. cinnamon powder

1 tsp. allspice

½ tsp. salt

Directions:

Set oven at 350F.

Bring the chia seeds in a small bowl then soak it with 6 tbsp. of water. Stir well and set aside.

In a mixing bowl, mix using a hand mixer the vegan butter and maple syrup until it turns fluffy. Add the chia seeds along with the mashed bananas.

Mix well and then add the coffee.

Meanwhile, sift all the dry ingredients (flour, baking powder, cinnamon powder, all spice, and salt) and then gradually add into the bowl with the wet ingredients.

Combine the ingredients well and then pour over a baking pan lined with parchment paper.

Place in the oven to bake for at least 30-40 minutes, or until the toothpick comes out clean after inserting in the bread.

Allow the bread to cool before serving.

Nutrition:

Calories: 371 kcal; Protein: 5.59 g; Fat: 16.81 g; Carbohydrates: 49.98 g

Instant Banana Oatmeal

Preparation Time: 1 minute

Cooking Time: 2 minutes

Servings: 1

Ingredients:

- 1 mashed ripe banana
- ½ c. water
- ½ c. quick oats

Directions:

Measure the oats and water into a microwave-safe bowl and stir to combine. Place bowl in microwave and heat on high for 2 minutes.

Remove bowl from microwave and stir in the mashed banana and enjoy.

Nutrition:

- ✓ Calories: 243 Cal
- ✓ Fat: 3 g
- ✓ Carbs: 50 g
- ✓ Protein: 6 g
- ✓ Sugars: 20 g

Almond Butter-Banana Smoothie

Preparation Time: 5 minutes

Cooking Time: 0

Servings: 1

Ingredients:

1 tbsp. almond butter

½ c. ice cubes

½ c. packed spinach

1 peeled and frozen medium banana

1 c. fat-free milk

Directions:

In a powerful blender, blend all ingredients until smooth and creamy.

Serve and enjoy.

Nutrition:

Calories: 293 Cal

Fat:9.8 g

Carbs:42.5 g

Protein:13.5 g

Sugars:12 g

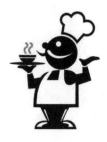

Brown Sugar Cinnamon Oatmeal

Preparation Time: 1 minute

Cooking Time: 3 minutes

Servings: 4

Ingredients:

½ tsp. ground cinnamon

1 ½ tsps. pure vanilla extract

¼ c. light brown sugar

2 c. low-fat milk

1 1/3 c. quick oats

Directions:

Measure the milk and vanilla into a medium saucepan and bring to a boil over medium-high heat.

Once boiling, reduce heat to medium. Stir in oats, brown sugar, and cinnamon, and cook, stirring, 2–3 minutes.

Serve immediately, sprinkled with additional cinnamon if desired.

Nutrition:

Calories: 208 Cal

Fat:3 g

Carbs:38 g

Protein:8 g

Sugars:15 g

Buckwheat Pancakes with Vanilla Almond Milk

Preparation Time: 10 minutes

Cooking Time: 4 minutes

Servings: 1

Ingredients:

½ c. unsweetened vanilla almond milk 2-4 packets natural sweetener

1/8 tsp. salt

½ cup buckwheat flour

½ tsp. double-acting baking powder

Directions:

Prepare a nonstick pancake griddle and spray with the cooking spray, place over medium heat.

Whisk together the buckwheat flour, salt, baking powder, and stevia in a small bowl and stir in the almond milk after.

Onto the pan, scoop a large spoonful of batter, cook until bubbles no longer pop on the surface and the entire surface looks dry and (2-4 minutes). Flip and cook for another 2-4 minutes. Repeat with all the remaining batter.

Nutrition:

Calories: 240 Cal

Fat:4.5 g

Carbs:2 g

Protein:11 g

Sugars:17 g

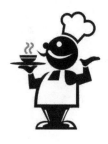

Tomato Bruschetta with Basil

Preparation Time: 10 minutes

Cooking Time: 0

Servings: 8

Ingredients:

½ c. chopped basil

2 minced garlic cloves

1 tbsp. balsamic vinegar

2 tbsps. Olive oil

½ tsp. cracked black pepper

1 sliced whole wheat baguette

8 diced ripe Roma tomatoes

1 tsp. sea salt

Directions:

First, preheat the oven to 375 F.

In a bowl, dice the tomatoes, mix in balsamic vinegar, chopped basil, garlic, salt, pepper, and olive oil, set aside.

Slice the baguette into 16-18 slices and for about 10 minutes, place on a baking pan to bake.

Serve with warm bread slices and enjoy.

For leftovers, store in an airtight container and put in the fridge. Try putting them over grilled chicken, it is amazing!

Nutrition:
Calories: 57 Cal

Fat:2.5 g

Carbs:7.9 g

Protein:1.4 g

Sugars:0.2 g

Mango Granola

Preparation Time: 10 minutes

Cooking Time: 30 minutes

Servings: 4

Ingredients:

2 cups rolled oats

1 cup dried mango, chopped

½ cup almonds, roughly chopped

½ cup nuts

½ cup dates, roughly chopped

3 tbsp. sesame seeds

2 tsp. cinnamon

2/3 cup agave nectar

2 tbsp. coconut oil

2 tbsp. water

Directions:

Set oven at 320F

In a large bowl, put the oats, almonds, nuts, sesame seeds, dates, and cinnamon then mix well.

Meanwhile, heat a saucepan over medium heat, pour in the agave syrup, coconut oil, and water.

Stir and let it cook for at least 3 minutes or until the coconut oil has melted.

Gradually pour the syrup mixture into the bowl with the oats and nuts and stir well, ensure that all the ingredients are coated with the syrup.

Transfer the granola on a baking sheet lined with parchment paper and place in the oven to bake for 20 minutes.

After 20 minutes, take off the tray from the oven and lay the chopped dried mango on top. Put back in the oven then bake again for another 5 minutes.

Let the granola cool to room temperature before serving or placing it in an airtight container for storage. The shelf life of the granola will last up to 2-3 weeks.

Nutrition:

Calories: 434 kcal; Protein: 13.16 g; Fat: 28.3 g; Carbohydrates: 55.19 g

Sautéed Veggies on Hot Bagels

Preparation Time: 10 minutes

Cooking Time: 16 minutes

Servings: 2

Ingredients:

1 yellow squash, diced

1 zucchini, sliced thin

½ onion, sliced thin

2 pcs. tomatoes, sliced

1 clove of garlic, chopped

salt and pepper to taste

1 tbsp. olive oil

2 pcs. vegan bagels

vegan butter for spread

Directions:

Heat the olive oil on the medium temperature in a cast-iron skillet.

Lower the heat to medium-low and sauté the onions for 10 minutes or until the onions start to brown.

Turn the heat again to medium and then add the diced squash and zucchini to the pan and cook for 5 minutes. Add the clove of garlic and cook for another minute.

Throw in the tomato slices to the pan and cook for 1 minute. Season with pepper and salt and turn off the heat.

Toast the bagels and cut in half.

Spread the bagels lightly with butter and serve with the sautéed veggies on top.

Nutrition:

Calories: 375 kcal

Protein: 14.69 g

Fat: 11.46 g

Carbohydrates: 54.61 g

Bake Apple Turnover

Preparation Time: 30 minutes
Cooking Time: 25 minutes
Servings: 4

Ingredients:

For the turnovers

4 apples, peeled, cored, diced into bite-sized pieces

1 Tbsp. almond flour

All-purpose flour, for rolling out the dough

1 frozen puff pastry, thawed

½ cup palm sugar, crumbled by hand to loosen granules

½ tsp. cinnamon powder

For the egg wash

1 egg white, whisked in

2 Tbsp. water

Directions:

For the filling: combine almond flour, cinnamon powder, and palm sugar until these resemble coarse meal. Toss in diced apples until well coated. Set aside.

On a lightly floured surface, roll the puff pastry until ¼ inch thin. Slice into 8 pieces of 4" x 4" squares.

Divide prepared apples into 8 equal portions. Spoon on individual puff pastry squares. Fold in half diagonally. Press edges to seal.
Place each filled pastry on a baking tray lined with parchment paper. Make sure there is ample space between pastries.

Freeze for at least 20 minutes, or till ready to bake.

Preheat oven to 400°F or 205°C for at 10 minutes.
Brush frozen pastries with egg wash. Bring in a hot oven, and cook for 12 to 15 minutes, or until these turn golden brown all over.
Take off the baking tray in the oven immediately. Cool slightly for easier handling. Place 1 apple turnover on a plate. Serve warm.

Nutrition:

Calories: 203 kcal; Protein: 5.29 g; Fat: 4.4 g; Carbohydrates: 38.25 g

Quinoa and Cauliflower Congee

Preparation Time: 10 minutes

Cooking Time:1 hour

Servings: 8

Ingredients:

1 cauliflower head, minced

2 tablespoons red quinoa

2 leeks, minced

1 tablespoon fresh ginger, grated

2 garlic cloves, grated

6 cups of water

2 tablespoons brown rice

1 tablespoon olive oil

1 tablespoon fish sauce

2 onions, minced

Pinch of white pepper

For Garnish

4 eggs, soft-boiled

2 red chilli, minced

1 lime, sliced into wedges

¼ cup packed basil leaves, torn

¼ cup loosely packed cilantro leaves, torn

¼ cup loosely packed spearmint leaves, torn

Directions:

Put olive oil into a huge skillet on medium heat. Sauté shallots, garlic, and ginger until limp and aromatic; pour into a slow cooker set at medium heat.

Except for garnishes, pour remaining ingredients into slow cooker; stir. Put the lid on. Cook for 6 hours. Turn off heat. Taste; adjust seasoning if needed.

Ladle congee into individual bowls. Garnish with basil leaves, cilantro leaves, red chilli, and spearmint leaves. Add 1 piece of soft-boiled egg on top of each; serve with a wedge of lime on the side. Slice egg just before eating so yolk runs into congee. Squeeze lime juice into congee just before eating.

Nutrition:

Calories: 138 kcal

Protein: 7.23 g

Fat: 7.65 g

Carbohydrates: 10.76 g

Breakfast Arrozcaldo

Preparation Time: 20 minutes

Cooking Time: 30 minutes

Servings: 5

Ingredients:

6 eggs, white only

1½ cups brown rice, cooked

For the filling

¼ cup raisins

½ cup frozen peas, thawed

1 white onion, minced

1 garlic clove, minced oil, for greasing

Directions:

For the filling, spray a small amount of oil into a skillet set over medium heat. Add in onion and garlic. Stir-fry until former is limp and transparent.

Stir-fry while breaking up clumps, about 2 minutes. Add in remaining ingredients. Stir-fry for another minute.

Turn down the heat, and let filling cook for 10 to 15 minutes, or until juices are greatly reduced. Stir often. Turn off heat. Divide into 6 equal portions.

For the eggs, spray a small amount of oil into a smaller skillet set over medium heat. Cook eggs. Discard yolk. Transfer to holding the plate.

To serve, place 1 portion of rice on a plate, 1 portion of filling, and 1 egg white. Serve warm.

Nutrition:

Calories: 53 kcal

Protein: 6.28 g

Fat: 1.35 g

Carbohydrates: 3.59 g

Apple Bruschetta with Almonds and Blackberries

Preparation Time: 20 minutes

Cooking Time: 30 minutes

Servings: 5

Ingredients:

1 apple, sliced into ¼-inch thick half-moons

¼ cup blackberries, thawed, lightly mashed ½ tsp. fresh lemon juice

⅛ cup almond slivers, toasted Sea salt

Directions:

Drizzle lemon juice on apple slices. Put these on a tray lined with parchment paper.

Spread a small number of mashed berries on top of each slice. Top these off with the desired amount of almond slivers.

Sprinkle sea salt on "bruschetta" just before serving.

Nutrition:

Calories: 56 kcal

Protein: 1.53 g

Fat: 1.43 g

Carbohydrates: 9.87 g

Chapter 3: Lunch

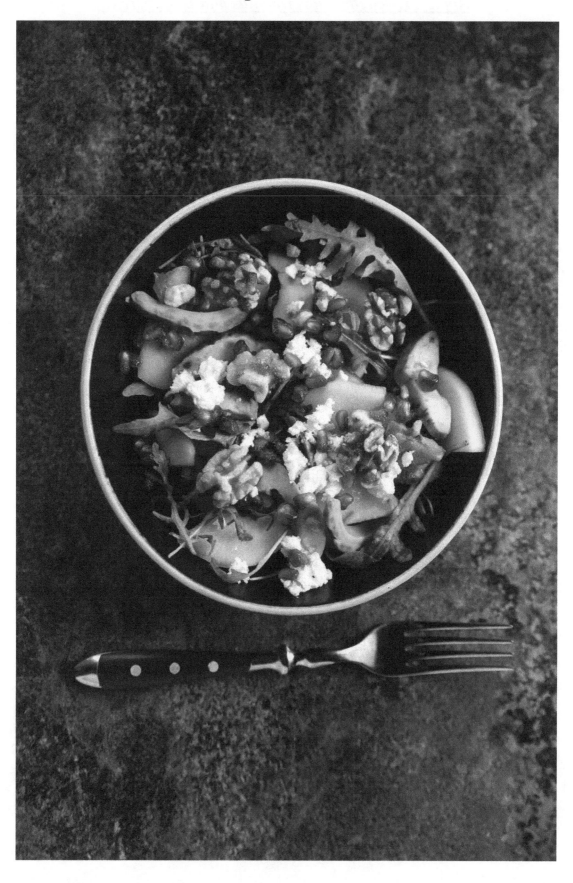

Greek Prosciutto-Wrapped Meatloaf

Preparation Time: 10 minutes
Cooking Time:50 minutes
Servings: 8

Ingredients:

2 teaspoons Greek seasoning blend

1/4 cup half-and-half

8 slices of prosciutto

1/2-pound ground lamb

2 eggs, beaten

1 tablespoon Worcester sauce

3 teaspoons olive oil

2 pounds ground beef

2 shallots, finely chopped

6 ounces feta cheese, crumbled

1 tablespoon brown mustard

1/2 cup chopped Kalamata olives

Directions:

Preheat your oven to a 3900F.

Heat the oil in a cast-iron skillet that is fore heated using a medium flame. Sauté the shallot until it gets soft and lightly browned.

In a large mixing container, completely merge the remaining ingredients, leaving out prosciutto. Add sautéed onion and stir well.

Shape the merge substance into a meatloaf. Wrap the meatloaf in the slices of prosciutto and move it to a baking pan.

Close it with a piece of aluminum foil. Bake for 40 minutes. Dispose of the foil and bake for an extra 10 to 13 minutes. Bon appétit!

Nutrition:

Calories: 442 Cal
Protein: 56.3 g
Fat: 20.6 g
Carbs: 4.9 g
Sugar: 1 g

Greek-Style Cold Beef Salad

Preparation Time: 15 minutes
Cooking Time: 3 minutes
Servings: 6

Ingredients:

- ✓ 1 orange bell pepper, thinly sliced
- ✓ 1 green bell pepper, thinly sliced
- ✓ 1 tablespoon fresh lemon juice
- ✓ Salt and ground black pepper, to your liking
- ✓ 1 cup grape tomatoes, halved
- ✓ 1 tablespoon soy sauce
- ✓ 1 ½ pounds beef rump steak
- ✓ 1/2 teaspoon dried oregano
- ✓ 1 head of butter lettuce, leaves separated
- ✓ 1 red onion, peeled and thinly sliced
- ✓ 2 cucumbers, thinly sliced
- ✓ 1/4 cup extra-virgin olive oil

Directions:

In a salad container, toss the onions, cucumbers, tomato, bell pepper, and butter lettuce leaves.

Fore heat a barbecue grill; heat the steak for 3 minutes per side. After that, thinly slice steak across the grain.
Include the slices of meat to the salad.

Prepare the dressing by whisking the oregano, salt, pepper, lemon juice, olive oil and soy sauce.

Dress the salad and enjoy well-chilled.

Nutrition:

- ✓ Calories: 315
- ✓ Protein: 37.5g
- ✓ Fat: 13.8g
- ✓ Carbs: 6.4g
- ✓ Sugar: 2.4g

Slow Cooked Chicken Curry

Preparation Time: 10 minutes

Cooking Time: 5 hours

Servings: 4

Ingredients:

2 sweet potatoes, cubed

3 chicken breasts, boneless, skinless and chopped

1 red bell pepper, chopped

1 small yellow onion, chopped
2 cups coconut milk

2 cups chicken stock

1 teaspoon ground cumin

3 tablespoons curry powder

2 tablespoons chopped cilantro

Salt and cayenne pepper to the taste

Directions:

In your slow cooker, mix the chicken the sweet potatoes, bell pepper, onion, stock, milk, cumin, curry powder, salt and cayenne. Cover and cook on Low for 5 hours then divide into bowls, sprinkle the cilantro on top and serve.

Enjoy!

Nutrition:

Calories: 280 Cal

Fat: 13 g

Fiber: 7 g

Carbs: 8 g

Protein: 15 g

Cumin Chicken Mix

Preparation Time: 2 hours

Cooking Time: 25 minutes

Servings: 4

Ingredients:

4 garlic cloves, minced

2 pounds chicken thighs, skinless and boneless

4 tablespoons extra-virgin olive oil

4 tablespoons chopped cilantro

2 tablespoons lime juice

A pinch of salt and black pepper

2 tablespoons olive oil

1 teaspoon cumin, ground

1 teaspoon red chili flakes

Lime wedges for serving

Directions:

In a bowl, whisk the olive oil with salt, pepper, cilantro, garlic, lime juice, cumin and chili flakes. Add the chicken, toss, cover and leave aside for 2 hours. Heat up a pan with the oil over medium-high heat, add chicken, cook for 3 minutes on each side and transfer to a baking dish. Cook in the oven at 375 degrees F for 20 minutes then divide between plates and serve with lime wedges on the side.

Enjoy!

Nutrition:

Calories: 200 Cal

Fat: 10 g

Fiber: 1 g

Carbs: 12 g

Protein: 24 g

Rosemary Chicken Thighs

Preparation Time: 10 minutes

Cooking Time: 40 minutes

Servings: 2

Ingredients:

14 ounces chicken thighs, bone-in

1 tablespoon lemon juice

1 teaspoon chili powder

A pinch of salt and black pepper

1 tablespoon fresh minced ginger

1 tablespoon olive oil

4 onions, chopped

2 rosemary springs, chopped

Directions:

In a bowl, mix chili powder with lemon juice and ginger. Add the chicken, rub it with this mix and then let sit for 10 minutes. Heat up a pan with the oil over medium-high heat, add the marinated chicken pieces and cook for 3 minutes on each side. Add rosemary, onions, salt and pepper. Reduce heat to medium, cover pan, cook for 25 minutes. Divide between plates and serve.

Enjoy!

Nutrition:

Calories 210 g

Fat 8 g

Fiber 9 g

Carbs 12 g

Protein 17 g

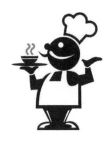

Turkey Stew

Preparation Time: 10 minutes

Cooking Time: 1 hour And 20 minutes

Servings: 6

Ingredients:

3 teaspoons olive oil

1 green bell pepper, chopped

1 pound ground turkey meat

1 tablespoons garlic, minced

1 yellow onion, chopped

1 teaspoon ground ancho chilies

1 tablespoon chili powder

2 teaspoons ground cumin

8 ounces canned green chilies and juice, chopped

8 ounces tomato paste

15 ounces canned tomatoes, chopped

2 cups veggie stock

A pinch of salt and black pepper

Directions:

Heat up a pan with 2 teaspoons oil over medium heat, add turkey, stir, brown well on all sides and transfer to a pot. Heat up the pan with the rest of the oil over medium heat and add onion and green bell pepper. Stir and cook for 3 minutes. Add garlic, chili powder, ancho chili powder, salt, pepper and cumin, stir and cook for 2 more minutes. Transfer this to the pot with the turkey meat, add chilies and juice, tomato sauce, chopped tomatoes, stock, salt and pepper. Stir, bring to a boil, cover the pot and cook for 1 hour. Divide into bowls and serve.

Enjoy!

Nutrition:
Calories: 327
Fat: 8
Fiber: 13
Carbs: 24
Protein: 27

Chicken and Mushroom Salad

Preparation Time: 10 minutes

Cooking Time: 0 minutes

Servings: 4

Ingredients:

1 yellow onion, chopped

12 ounces canned mushrooms, drained and chopped

2 garlic cloves, minced

2 teaspoons chopped rosemary

3 cups chicken, already cooked and shredded

2 cups baby spinach

Salt and black pepper to the tastes

A splash of balsamic vinegar

A drizzle of olive oil

Directions:

In a bowl, mix the mushrooms with the chicken, onion, garlic, rosemary, spinach, salt, pepper, vinegar and oil, toss and serve.

Enjoy!

Nutrition:

Calories: 210 Cal

Fat: 5 g

Fiber: 8 g

Carbs: 15 g

Protein:11 g

Shrimp Cakes

Preparation Time: 10 minutes

Cooking Time: 10 minutes

Servings: 24

Ingredients:

½ pound tiger shrimp, peeled, deveined and chopped A pinch of sea salt and black pepper

2 tablespoons olive oil
½ pound ground pork

1 egg, whisked

2 tablespoons coconut flour

2 tablespoons chicken stock

1 teaspoon coconut aminos

1 green onion stalk, chopped

1 teaspoon fresh grated ginger Directions:

In a bowl, mix the shrimp with the pork, salt, pepper, egg, stock, aminos, onion, ginger and flour. Stir well and shape medium cakes out of this mix. Heat up a pan with the oil over medium-high heat, add the cakes and cook for 5 minutes on each side. Divide between plates and serve with a side salad.

Enjoy!

Nutrition:

Calories 281 Cal

Fat 8 g

Fiber 7 g

Carbs 19 g

Protein 8 g

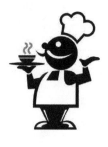

Italian Calamari

Preparation Time: 10 minutes

Cooking Time: 30 minutes

Servings: 6

Ingredients:

15 ounces canned tomatoes, chopped

1 ½ pounds calamari, cleaned, tentacles separated and cut into thin strips

1 garlic clove, minced

½ cup veggie stock

1 bunch chopped parsley

A pinch red pepper flakes

Juice of lemon

A drizzle of olive oil

A pinch of sea salt and black pepper

Directions:

Heat up a pan with the oil over medium-high heat, add the garlic and pepper flakes, stir and cook for 2-3 minutes. Add calamari, stir and cook for 3 minutes more. Add tomatoes, stock, lemon juice, salt and pepper, bring to a simmer then reduce heat to medium and cook for 25 minutes. Add the parsley, stir, divide into bowls and serve.

Enjoy!

Nutrition:

Calories 228 Cal

Fat 2 g

Fiber 4 g

Carbs 11 g

Protein 39 g

Chili Snapper

Preparation Time: 10 minutes

Cooking Time: 20 minutes

Servings: 2

Ingredients:

2 red snapper fillets, boneless and skinless

3 tablespoons chili paste

A pinch of sea salt and black pepper

1 tablespoon coconut aminos

1 garlic clove, minced

½ teaspoon fresh grated ginger

2 teaspoons sesame seeds, toasted

2 tablespoons olive oil

1 green onion, chopped

2 tablespoons chicken stock

Directions:

Heat up a pan with the oil over medium-high heat, add the ginger, onion and the garlic, stir and cook for 2 minutes. Add chili paste, aminos, salt, pepper and the stock, stir and cook for 3 minutes more. Add the fish fillets, toss gently and cook for 5-6 minutes on each side. Divide between plates, sprinkle sesame seeds on top and serve.

Enjoy!

Nutrition:

Calories 261

Fat: 10 g

Fiber: 7 g

Carbs: 15 g

Protein:16 g

Thai Cod

Preparation Time: 10 minutes

Cooking Time: 10 minutes

Servings: 2

Ingredients:

1 tablespoon coconut aminos

1 cup coconut milk

1 tablespoon Thai curry paste

A drizzle of olive oil

Zest of 1 lime

Juice of ½ lime

1 tablespoon fresh grated ginger

1 teaspoon garlic, minced

2 cod fillets, boneless

1 tablespoon chopped cilantro

Directions:

In a bowl, whisk the aminos with coconut cream, curry paste, lime zest and juice, ginger and garlic. Add the cod, toss to cover and set aside for 10 minutes to marinate. Heat up a pan with a drizzle of oil over medium heat, add the cod, cook for 5 minutes on each side, divide between plates and sprinkle cilantro on top then serve.

Enjoy!

Nutrition:

Calories: 271 Cal

Fat 4 g

Fiber 6 g

Carbs 14 g

Protein 7 g

Tarragon Chicken with Roasted Balsamic Turnips

Preparation Time: 10 minutes

Cooking Time: 50 minutes

Servings: 2-4

Ingredients:

1 pound chicken thighs

2 lb. turnips, cut into wedges

2 tbsp. olive oil

1 tbsp. balsamic vinegar

1 tbsp. tarragon

Salt and black pepper, to taste

Directions:

Set the oven to 400°F then grease a baking dish with olive oil. Cook turnips in boiling water for 10 minutes, drain and set aside. Add the chicken and turnips to the baking dish.
Sprinkle with tarragon, black pepper, and salt. Roast for 35 minutes. Remove the baking dish, drizzle the turnip wedges with balsamic vinegar and return to the oven for another 5 minutes.

Nutrition:

Calories: 383

Fat: 26g

Net Carbs: 9.5g

Protein: 21.3g

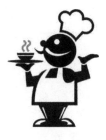

Tomato & Cheese Chicken Chili

Preparation Time: 5 minutes

Cooking Time: 25 minutes

Servings: 2-4

Ingredients:

1 tbsp. butter

1 tbsp. olive oil

1 pound chicken breasts, skinless, boneless, cubed

½ onion, chopped

2 cups chicken broth

2 cups tomatoes, chopped

2 oz. tomato puree

1 tbsp. chili powder

1 tbsp. cumin

1 garlic clove, minced

1 habanero pepper, minced

½ cup mozzarella cheese, shredded

Salt and black pepper to taste

Directions:

Season the chicken using salt and pepper. Set a large pan at medium heat and add the chicken; cover it with water, and bring it to a boil. Cook until no longer pink, for 10 minutes.

Transfer the chicken to a flat surface to shred with forks. In a pot, pour in the butter and olive oil and set over medium heat. Sauté onion and garlic until transparent for 5 minutes.

Stir in the chicken, tomatoes, cumin, habanero pepper, tomato puree, broth, and chili powder. Adjust the seasoning and let the mixture boil.

Reduce heat to simmer for about 10 minutes. Top with shredded cheese to serve.

Nutrition:

Calories: 322

Fat: 16.6g

Net Carbs: 6.2g

Protein: 29g

Turmeric Chicken Wings with Ginger Sauce

Preparation Time: 5 minutes

Cooking Time: 20 minutes

Servings: 2-4

Ingredients:

2 tbsp. olive oil

1 pound chicken wings, cut in half

1 tbsp. turmeric

1 tbsp. cumin

3 tbsp. fresh ginger, grated

Salt and black pepper, to taste

Juice of ½ lime

1 cup thyme leaves

¾ cup cilantro, chopped

1 tbsp. water

1 jalapeño pepper Directions:

In a bowl, stir together 1 tbsp. ginger, cumin, and salt, half of the olive oil, black pepper, turmeric, and cilantro. Place in the chicken wings pieces, toss to coat, and refrigerate for 20 minutes.

Heat the grill to high heat. Remove the wings from the marinade, drain, and grill for 20 minutes, turning from time to time, then set aside.

Using a blender, combine thyme, remaining ginger, salt, jalapeno pepper, black pepper, lime juice, the remaining olive oil, and water, and blend well. Serve the chicken wings topped with the sauce.

Nutrition:

Calories 253

Fat 16.1g

Net Carbs 4.1g

Protein 21.7g

Feta & Bacon Chicken

Preparation Time: 20 minutes

Cooking Time: 10minutes

Servings: 2-4

Ingredients:

4 oz. bacon, chopped

1 pound chicken breasts

3 green onions, chopped

2 tbsp. coconut oil

4 oz. feta cheese, crumbled

1 tbsp. parsley

Directions:

Place a pan over medium heat and coat with cooking spray. Add in the bacon and cook until crispy. Remove to paper towels, drain the grease and crumble.

To the same pan, add in the oil and cook the chicken breasts for 4-5 minutes, then flip to the other side; cook for an additional 4-5 minutes. Place the chicken breasts to a baking dish. Place the green onions, set in the oven, turn on the broiler, and cook for 5 minutes at high temperature. Remove to serving plates and serve topped with bacon, feta cheese, and parsley.

Nutrition:

Calories 459

Fat 35g

Net Carbs 3.1g

Protein 31.5g

Chicken Pie with Bacon

Preparation Time: 20 minutes
Cooking Time: 35 minutes
Servings: 24

Ingredients:

3 tbsp. butter

1 onion, chopped

4 oz. bacon, sliced

1 carrot, chopped

3 garlic cloves, minced

Salt and black pepper, to taste

¾ cup crème fraiche

¾ ½ cup chicken stock

1 pound chicken breasts, cubed

2 tbsp. yellow mustard

¾ cup cheddar cheese, shredded Dough

1 egg

¾ cup almond flour

3 tbsp. cream cheese

1 ½ cups mozzarella cheese, shredded

1 tsp onion powder

1 tsp garlic powder

Salt and black pepper, to taste

Directions:

Sauté the onion, garlic, black pepper, bacon, and carrot in melted butter for 5 minutes. Add in the chicken and cook for 3 minutes. Stir in the crème fraîche, salt, mustard, black pepper, and stock, and cook for 7 minutes. Add in the cheddar cheese and set aside.

In a bowl, combine the mozzarella cheese with the cream cheese and heat in a microwave for 1 minute. Stir in the garlic powder, salt, flour, black pepper, onion powder, and egg. Knead the dough well, split into 4 pieces, and flatten each into a circle.

Set the chicken mixture into 4 ramekins, top each with a dough circle, and cook in the oven at 370 F for 25 minutes.

Nutrition:

Calories 563

Fat 44.6g
Net Carbs 7.7g

Protein 36g

Flying Jacob Casserole

Preparation Time: 15 minutes
Cooking Time: 20-25 minutes
Servings: 6

Ingredients:

1 pc Grilled Chicken

2 tbsp. Butter

225 g Diced bacon

250 g Mushrooms

475 ml Cream

125 ml hot chili sauce

1 tsp. Seasoning curry

Salt and black pepper to taste

125 g Peanuts

Salad

175 g Spinach

2 pcs Tomato

Directions:

Preheat the oven to 400 ° F.

Chop the mushrooms into small pieces then fry in oil with bacon. Salt and pepper to taste.

Separate the chicken meat from the bones and chop it into small pieces.

Put these pieces of chicken in a mold for baking, oiled. Add mushrooms and bacon.

Beat the cream until soft peaks. Put chili sauce, curry, and salt and pepper to taste.

Pour the chicken into the resulting mixture.

Bake in the oven for at least 20-25 minutes until the dish will get a pleasant golden color.
Sprinkle toasted and chopped nuts on top. Serve with salad.

Nutrition:

Carbohydrates: 11 g
Fats: 80 g
Proteins: 40 g
Calories: 912

BBQ Chicken Zucchini Boats

Preparation Time: 10 minutes
Cooking Time: 15-20 minutes
Servings: 4

Ingredients:

3 Zucchini halved

1 lb. cooked Chicken breast

.5 cup BBQ sauce

.33 cup Shredded Mexican cheese

1 Avocado, sliced

.5 cup Halved cherry tomatoes

.25 cup Diced green onions

3 tbsp. Keto-friendly ranch dressing

Also Needed: 9x13 casserole dish

Directions:

Set the oven to reach 350° Fahrenheit.

Using a knife, cut the zucchini in half. Discard the seeds. Make the boat by carving out of the center. Place the zucchini flesh side up into the casserole dish.

Discard and cut the skin and bones from the chicken. Shred and add the chicken in with the barbeque sauce. Toss to coat all the chicken fully.

Fill the zucchini boats with the mixture using about .25 to .33 cup each.

Sprinkle with Mexican cheese on top.

Bake for approximately 15 minutes. (If you would like it tenderer; bake for an additional 5 to 10 minutes to reach the desired tenderness.)

Remove from the oven. Top it off with avocado, green onion, tomatoes, and a drizzle of dressing. Serve.

Nutrition:

Calories: 212

Net Carbs: 9 g

Total Fat Content: 11 g

Protein: 19 g

Creamy Chicken & Greens

Preparation Time: 10 minutes

Cooking Time: 20 minutes

Servings: 4

Ingredients:

1 lb. Chicken thighs – skins on

1 cup. Chicken stock

1 cup. Cream

2 tbsp. Coconut oil

1 tsp. Italian herbs

2 cups Dark leafy greens

Pepper & Salt (your preference)

2 tbsp. Coconut flour

2 tbsp. Melted butter

Directions:

On the stovetop, add oil in a skillet using the med-high temperature setting.

Remove the bones from the chicken and dust using salt and pepper. Fry the chicken until done.

Make the sauce by adding the butter to a saucepan. Whisk in the flour to form a thick paste. Slowly, whisk in the cream. Once it boils, mix in the herbs.

Transfer the chicken to the counter and add the stock.

Deglaze the pan, and whisk the cream sauce. Toss in the greens until thoroughly coated with the sauce.

Arrange the thighs on the greens, warm up, and serve.

Nutrition:

Calories: 446

Net Carbs: 3 g

Total Fat Content: 38 g

Protein: 18 g

Cod and Peas

Preparation Time: 10 minutes

Cooking Time: 15 minutes

Servings: 4

Ingredients:

10 ounces peas, blanched

1 tablespoon chopped parsley

A drizzle of olive oil

4 cod fillets, boneless

1 teaspoon dried oregano

2 ounces veggie stock

2 garlic cloves, minced

1 teaspoon smoked paprika

A pinch of sea salt and black pepper

Directions:

Put parsley, paprika, oregano, stock and garlic in your food processor and blend really well. Heat up a pan with the oil over medium-high heat, add the cod, season with salt and pepper and cook for 4 minutes on each side. Add the peas and the parsley, mix and cook for 5 minutes more. Divide everything between plates and serve.

Enjoy!

Nutrition:

Calories: 271 Cal

Fat: 4 g

Fiber: 6 g

Carbs: 14 g

Protein: 15 g

Salmon and Scallions

Preparation Time: 10 minutes

Cooking Time: 20 minutes

Servings: 4

Ingredients:

4 medium salmon fillets, boneless

4 scallions, chopped

2 tablespoons olive oil
Zest of 1 lemon

1 teaspoon white vinegar

¼ cup chopped dill

¼ cup chicken stock

A pinch of sea salt and black pepper

Directions:

Heat up a pan with half of the oil over medium-high heat, add the salmon, season with salt and pepper then cook for 6 minutes on each side and divide between plates. Heat up another pan with the rest of the oil over medium-high heat. Add scallions, stir and cook for 2 minutes. Add lemon zest, vinegar, dill, stock, salt and pepper. Stir and cook for 5 minutes more, pour over the salmon and serve.

Enjoy!

Nutrition:

Calories 300 Cal

Fat: 4 g

Fiber: 8 g

Carbs: 14 g

Protein: 17 g

Salmon and Carrots

Preparation Time: 10 minutes

Cooking Time: 15 minutes

Servings: 2

Ingredients:

1 tablespoon ground cinnamon

2 tablespoon olive oil

2 salmon fillets, bone-in

2 cups baby carrots

1 tablespoon lime juice

A pinch of sea salt and black pepper

Directions:

In a bowl, mix the cinnamon with half of the oil, salt and pepper then rub the salmon with this mix. Place the salmon on the preheated grill over medium-high heat, cook for 5 minutes on each side and divide between plates. Heat up a pan with the rest of the oil over medium-high heat and add the carrots, lime juice, salt and pepper. Toss and cook for 5-6 minutes then divide next to the salmon and serve.
Enjoy!

Nutrition:

Calories: 371

Fat: 26

Fiber: 2

Carbs: 6

Protein: 22

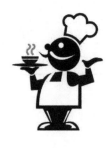

Chinese Mackerel

Preparation Time: 10 minutes

Cooking Time: 30 minutes

Servings: 4

Ingredients:

1 garlic clove, minced

1 shallot, chopped

1 cup chicken stock

2 pounds mackerel, skinless, boneless and cubed

1 small ginger piece, chopped

1 yellow onion, chopped

2 celery stalks, chopped

1 teaspoon hot mustard

1 tablespoon rice vinegar

A pinch of black pepper

A drizzle of olive oil

Directions:

Heat up a pan with the oil over medium-high heat, add the mackerel, season with black pepper and cook for 4 minutes. Add the garlic, shallot, onion, ginger and celery, toss and cook for 4 minutes more, flipping the fish as well. Add stock, mustard and vinegar, toss gently and cook for 20 minutes over medium heat. Divide into bowls and serve.

Enjoy!

Nutrition:

Calories: 261 Cal

Fat: 4 g

Fiber: 8 g

Carbs: 14 g

Protein: 7 g

Lemony Mackerel

Preparation Time: 10 minutes

Cooking Time: 15 minutes

Servings: 4

Ingredients:

Juice of 1 lemon

Zest of 1 lemon

4 mackerels

1 tablespoon minced chives

A pinch of sea salt and black pepper

2 tablespoons olive oil

Directions:

Heat up a pan with the oil over medium-high heat, add the mackerel and cook for 6 minutes on each side. Add the lemon zest, lemon juice, chives, salt and pepper then cook for 2 more minutes on each side. Divide everything between plates and serve.

Enjoy!

Nutrition:

Calories: 289 Cal

Fat :20 g

Fiber: 0 g

Carbs: 1 g

Protein: 21 g

Chapter 4: Dinner

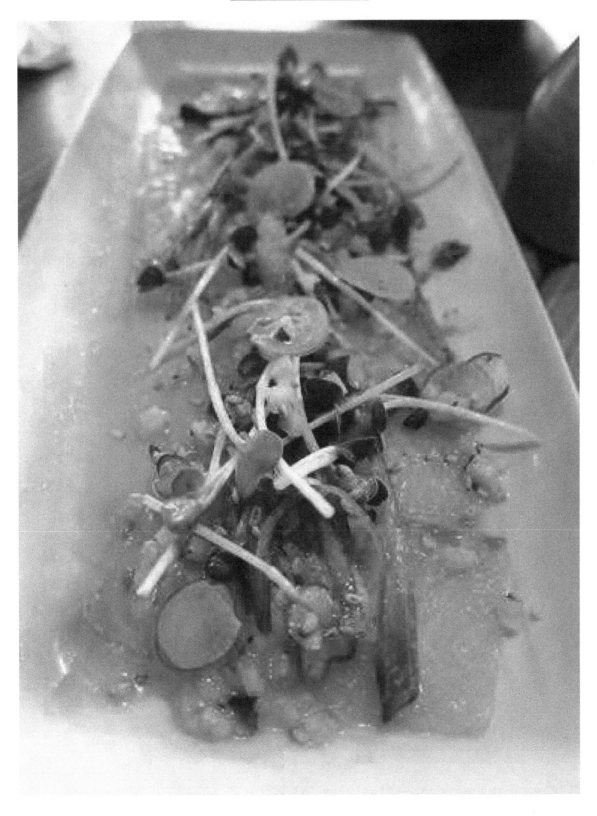

Grilled Beef Angus and Chorizo

Preparation Time: 10 minutes

Cooking Time: 20 minutes

Servings: 2

Ingredients:

- ✓ 1 lb. High River Angus, in thin steaks
- ✓ One bottle of 12 oz. of Mexican beer, use Pacifico, Sol or Montejo
- ✓ One teaspoon salt
- ✓ 1 Smoky Ridge
- ✓ One medium white onion
- ✓ 1 ½ pepper red peppers (paprika)
- ✓ One tablespoon of olive oil or canola
- ✓ One teaspoon garlic salt
- ✓ Pepper to taste
- ✓ One package of 24 tortillas taquerias, if you want to serve the tacos with double tortilla, you will need two packages.
- ✓ Red sauce, green sauce, or avocado sauce
- ✓ Ten small lemons, optional

Directions:

In a bowl place the steaks, beer and a spoonful of salt. Cover put in refrigerator and marina for 1 hour.

Peel the chorizo and chop it into small pieces. Leave aside.

Chop the onion and chili peppers finely.

Heat the vegetable oil in the skillet and fry the onion until it softens about 2 minutes. Add the chopped peppers and cook, occasionally stirring for about 5 minutes or until the peppers are softened.

Heat a rotisserie to cook the chopped sausage for about 5 minutes or until it is fully cooked.

Smoke the steaks one by one, depending on how thick it will take about two minutes per side. Slice the roasted steaks into thin strips.

Stir in steaks and chorizo. Add the vegetables, garlic salt, and pepper to taste. Cook for two more minutes. Adjust salt.

Serve in tacos accompanied by the sauce of your liking and lemon juice, if you wish.

Nutrition:
Energy (calories): 875 kcal

Protein: 65.44 g

Fat: 64.38 g

Carbohydrates: 6.81 g

Fruits With Caramel Sauce

Preparation Time: 10 minutes

Cooking time: 30 to 60 min

Servings: 4

Ingredients:

For the fruit kebabs:

2 apples

1 mango

1/2 pineapple

8 strawberries 1/2 lemon

1 tbsp. sugar for the caramel sauce:

150 g butter

70 g of sugar

100 ml whipped cream

Directions:

Peel the apples for the grilled fruit, cut into slices, removing the core casing. Peel the mango, remove the core and cut into slices or cubes. Peel the pineapple, remove the woody interior and cut into cubes. Wash the strawberries, remove leaf green.

Squeeze out the lemon. Sprinkle the fruit with lemon juice and sprinkle with sugar. Alternately place the pieces of fruit on electric smoker, turning frequently. Melt the butter and brush the fruit skewers with the melted butter over and over while grilling.

For the caramel sauce, put butter and sugar in a saucepan and melt. Stir till the sugar become dissolved and it turned brown. Heat whipped cream in electric smoker and stir in the caramel.

The grilled fruits serve with caramel sauce.

Nutrition:

Energy (calories): 789 kcal

Protein: 1.61 g

Fat: 61.33 g

Carbohydrates: 65.22 g

Eggplant Cannelloni

Preparation Time: 10 minutes
Cooking Time: 20 minutes
Servings: 2

Ingredients:

1 Eggplant

2 tuna cans

1 Cooked egg Ground pepper Healthy tomato sauce

Grated Eat lean Protein Cheese

Directions:

Preheat your electric smoker to 225˚F.

We wash the eggplant well, we cut the ends and with the help of a mandolin we laminate it.

Now we are going to crush the 2 cans of tuna with the boiled egg to create the filling of the cannelloni.

Once we have all the ingredients prepared we will start making our rolls.

We put a little bit of the mixture in the widest point of the eggplant and we roll until the end.

We close with the help of a toothpick.

Repeat the operation until finishing with the filling.

Now we place all our cannelloni in a mold suitable for the electric smoker.

Season with pepper to taste.

We put a teaspoon of tomato on top.

And we finished with a little bit of low fat cheese.

Bake at 200º for 20-30min (depending on the electric smoker) Ready! We already have our aubergine cannelloni

Nutrition:

Energy (calories): 264 kcal

Protein: 38.34 g

Fat: 5.54 g

Carbohydrates: 18.43 g

Pork with Chili Zucchinis and Tomatoes

Preparation Time: 10 minutes
Cooking Time: 35 minutes
Servings: 4

Ingredients:

2 tomatoes, cubed

2 pounds pork stew meat, cubed

4 scallions, chopped

2 tablespoons olive oil

1 zucchini, sliced

Juice of 1 lime

2 tablespoons chili powder

½ tablespoons cumin powder Pinch of sea salt

Pinch black pepper

Directions:

Warm a pan with the oil on medium heat, add the scallions and sauté for 5 minutes. Add the meat and brown for 5 minutes more.

Add the tomatoes and the other ingredients, toss, cook over medium heat for 25 minutes more, divide between plates and serve.

Nutrition:

Calories 300

Fat 5

Fiber 2

Carbs 12

Protein 14

Pork with Thyme Sweet Potatoes

Preparation Time: 10 minutes
Cooking Time: 35 minutes
Servings: 4

Ingredients:

2 sweet potatoes, cut into wedges

4 pork chops

3 spring onions, chopped

1 tablespoon thyme, chopped
2 tablespoons olive oil

4 garlic cloves, minced

Pinch of sea salt

Pinch black pepper

½ cup vegetable stock

½ tablespoon chives, chopped

Directions:

In a roasting pan, combine the pork chops with the potatoes and the other ingredients, toss gently and cook at 390 degrees F for 35 minutes.

Divide everything between plates and serve.

Nutrition:

Calories 210

Fat 12.2

Fiber 5.2

Carbs 12

Protein 10

Pork with Pears and Ginger

Preparation Time: 10 minutes

Cooking Time: 35 minutes

Servings: 4

Ingredients:

2 green onions, chopped

2 tablespoons avocado oil

2 pounds pork roast, sliced

½ cup coconut aminos

1 tablespoon ginger, minced

2 pears, cored and cut into wedges

¼ cup vegetable stock

1 tablespoon chives, chopped

Directions:

Warm a pan with the oil on medium heat, add the onions, and the meat and brown for 2 minutes on each side.

Add the rest of the ingredients, toss gently, and bake at 390 degrees F for 30 minutes.

Divide the mix between plates and serve.

Nutrition:

Calories 220

Fat 13.3

Fiber 2

Carbs 16.5

Protein 8

Parsley Pork and Artichokes

Preparation Time: 10 minutes
Cooking Time: 35 minutes
Servings: 4

Ingredients:

2 tbsp. balsamic vinegar

1 cup canned artichoke hearts, drained

2 tbsp. olive oil

2 lb. pork stew meat, cubed

2 tbsp. parsley, chopped

1 tsp. cumin, ground

1 tsp. turmeric powder

2 garlic cloves, minced

Pinch of sea salt

Pinch black pepper

Directions:

Warm a pan with the oil on medium heat, add the meat and brown for 5 minutes.

Add the artichokes, the vinegar, and the other ingredients, toss, cook over medium heat for 30 minutes, divide between plates and serve.

Nutrition:

Calories 260

Fat 5

Fiber 4

Carbs 11

Protein 20

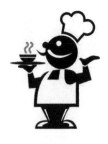

Pork with Mushrooms and Cucumbers

Preparation Time: 10 minutes
Cooking Time: 25 minutes
Servings: 4

Ingredients:

2 tablespoons olive oil

½ teaspoon oregano, dried

4 pork chops

2 garlic cloves, minced Juice of 1 lime

¼ cup cilantro, chopped Pinch of sea salt Pinch black pepper

1 cup white mushrooms, halved

2 tablespoons balsamic vinegar

Directions:

Warm a pan with the oil on medium heat, add the pork chops and brown for 2 minutes on each side.

Put the rest of the ingredients, toss, cook on medium heat for 20 minutes, divide between plates and serve.

Nutrition:

Calories 220

Fat 6

Fiber 8

Carbs 14.2

Protein 20

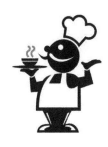

Oregano Pork

Preparation Time: 10 minutes

Cooking Time: 8 hours

Servings: 4

Ingredients:

2 pounds pork roast, sliced

2 tablespoons oregano, chopped

¼ cup balsamic vinegar
1 cup tomato paste

1 tablespoon sweet paprika

1 teaspoon onion powder

2 tablespoons chili powder

2 garlic cloves, minced

A pinch of salt and black pepper

Directions:

In your slow cooker, combine the roast with the oregano, the vinegar, and the other ingredients, toss, put the lid on and cook on Low for 8 hours.

Divide everything between plates and serve.

Nutrition:

Calories 300

Fat 5

Fiber 2

Carbs 12,

Protein 24

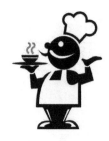

Curry Chicken Lettuce Wraps

Preparation Time: 15 minutes

Cooking Time: 10 minutes

Servings: 5

Ingredients:

2 Minced garlic cloves

.25 cups Minced onion

1 lb. Chicken thighs – skinless & boneless

2 tbsp. Ghee

1 tsp. Black pepper

2 tsp. Curry powder

1.5 tsp. Salt

1 cup Riced cauliflower

5-6 Lettuce leaves

Keto-friendly sour cream (as desired - count the carbs)

Directions:

Mince the garlic and onions. Set aside for now.
Pull out the bones and skin from the chicken and dice into one-inch pieces.

On the stovetop, add 2 tbsp. of ghee to a skillet and melt. Toss in the onion and sauté until browned. Fold in the chicken and sprinkle with the garlic, pepper, and salt.

Cook for eight minutes. Stir in the remainder of the ghee, riced cauliflower, and curry. Stir until well mixed.

Prepare the lettuce leaves and add the mixture.

Serve with a dollop of cream.

Nutrition:

Calories: 554

Net Carbs: 7 g

Total Fat Content: 36 g

Protein: 50 g

Nacho Chicken Casserole

Preparation Time: 15 minutes
Cooking Time: 25 minutes
Servings: 6
Ingredients:

1 medium Jalapeño pepper

1.75lb. Chicken thighs

Pepper and salt (to taste)

2 tbsp. Olive oil

1.5tsp. Chili seasoning

4 oz. Cheddar cheese

4 oz. Cream cheese

3 tbsp. Parmesan cheese

1 cup Green chilies and tomatoes

.25 cup Sour cream

1 pkg. Frozen cauliflower

Also Needed: Immersion blender

Directions:

Warm the oven to reach 375° Fahrenheit.

Slice the jalapeño into pieces and set aside.

Cutaway the skin and bones from the chicken. Chop it and sprinkle using the pepper and salt. Prepare in a skillet using a portion of olive oil on the med-high temperature setting until browned.

Mix in the sour cream, cream cheese, and ¾ of the cheddar cheese. Stir until melted and combined well. Place in the tomatoes and chilies. Stir then put it all to a baking dish.

Cook the cauliflower in the microwave. Blend in the rest of the cheese with the immersion blender until it resembles mashed potatoes. Season as desired.

Spread the cauliflower concoction over the casserole and sprinkle with the peppers. Bake approximately 15 to 20 minutes.

Nutrition:

Calories: 426
Net Carbs: 4.3 g
Total Fat Content: 32.2 g
Protein: 31 g

Pesto & Mozzarella Chicken Casserole

Preparation Time: 10 minutes

Cooking Time: 25-30 minutes

Servings: 8

Ingredients:

Cooking oil (as needed)

2 lb. Grilled & cubed chicken breasts

8 oz. Cubed mozzarella

8 oz. Cream cheese

8 oz. Shredded mozzarella

.25 cup Pesto

.25 to .5 cup Heavy cream

Directions:

Warm the oven to 400º Fahrenheit. Spritz a casserole dish with a spritz of cooking oil spray.

Combine the pesto, heavy cream, and softened cream cheese.

Add the chicken and cubed mozzarella into the greased dish.

Sprinkle the chicken using the shredded mozzarella. Bake for 25-30 minutes.

Nutrition:

Calories: 451

Net Carbs: 3 g

Total Fat Content: 30 g

Protein: 38 g

Spicy Habanero and Ground Beef Dinner

Preparation Time: 10 minutes

Cooking Time: 30 minutes

Servings: 2

Ingredients:

- ✓ 1/2 teaspoon ground black pepper
- ✓ 1/2 teaspoon dried thyme
- ✓ 1/2 teaspoon dried basil
- ✓ 1 ½ pounds ground chuck
- ✓ 1 teaspoon habanero pepper, minced
- ✓ 1/2 teaspoon ground bay leaf
- ✓ 2 tablespoons tallow, at room temperature
- ✓ 2 ripe Roma tomatoes, crushed
- ✓ 2 shallots, chopped
- ✓ 1 teaspoon fennel seeds
- ✓ 2 garlic cloves, minced
- ✓ 1/4 teaspoon caraway seeds, ground
- ✓ 1/2 cup dry sherry wine
- ✓ 1/2 teaspoon paprika
- ✓ 1/2 teaspoon salt
- ✓ For Ketogenic Tortillas:
- ✓ A pinch of table salt
- ✓ 4 egg whites
- ✓ A pinch of Swerve
- ✓ 1/3 teaspoon baking powder
- ✓ 1/4 cup coconut flour
- ✓ 6 tablespoons water

Directions:

Dissolve the tallow in a wok that is forehead over a normal high heat.

Following the above step, brown the ground chuck for 4 minutes, breaking it with a fork. Include all seasonings along with garlic, shallots, and habanero pepper. After that, keep on cooking for an additional 9 minutes.

Succeeding the above step, stir in the tomatoes and sherry. Then adjust the heat to medium-low, shut the lid, and let it simmer for a longer period of 20 minutes.

In the meantime, prepare the tortillas by mixing the coconut flour, eggs, and baking powder in a container. Add together the salt, water, and Swerve, then mix until everything is well included.

Foreheat a nonstick skillet with a moderate flame. Bake tortillas for a notable time on each side.

Again, repeat until there is no more batter.

Enjoy ground beef mixture.

Nutrition:

Calories: 361 Cal

Protein: 29 g

Fat: 21.9 g

Carbs: 6.4 g

Sugar: 1.5 g

Meatballs with Roasted Peppers and Manchego

Preparation Time: 10 minutes

Cooking Time 50 minutes

Servings: 2

Ingredients:

2 leeks, chopped

2 ripe tomatoes, crushed

1 pound ground beef

1 teaspoon lemon thyme

3 garlic cloves

1 egg

3 tablespoons parmesan cheese, grated

1 ½ cups chicken broth

1/2 teaspoon fresh ginger, ground

4 bell peppers, deveined and chopped

2 chipotle peppers, deveined and minced

1/2 cup Manchego cheese, crumbled

Salt and freshly ground black pepper

Directions:

Heat- Broil the peppers for about 20 minutes while turning once or twice). Permit them to stand for about a minimum of 30 minutes to loosen the skin.

Skin the peppers; get rid of stems and seeds; slice chipotle peppers into equal parts and reserve.

In a mixing dish, merge the parmesan, leeks, egg, garlic, salt, pepper, and ground beef. Cook a heavy-bottomed skillet over moderately high heat.

Brown meatballs on all sides for about 10 minutes.

After the above step, make the tomato sauce. Cook the tomatoes, ginger, chicken broth, and lemon thyme in a pan that is preheated over medium-high heat; spice with salt and pepper to taste.

Enable it to boil, reduce the heat to medium. Add meatballs and let them simmer until they are completely cooked, careful stirring.

Serve meatballs with the tomato sauce and roasted peppers. Garnish with crumbled Manchego and serve!

Nutrition:

Calories: 348 Cal; Protein: 42.8 g; Fat: 13.7 g; Carbs: 5.9 g; Sugar: 2.7 g

The Best Sloppy Joes Ever

Preparation Time: 10 minutes

Cooking Time: 20 minutes

Servings: 6

Ingredients:

1 teaspoon deli mustard

Salt and ground pepper, to taste

1 ½ pounds ground chuck

2 teaspoons tallow, room temperature

2 shallots, finely chopped

1 tablespoon coconut vinegar

1 teaspoon chipotle powder

1 teaspoon celery seeds

1/2 cup pureed tomatoes

1 teaspoon garlic, minced

1 teaspoon cayenne pepper

Directions:

Dissolve 1 tablespoon of tallow in a heavy-bottomed skillet using a normal high flame.

After the above, sauté the shallots and garlic till they become tender and aromatic; reserve. In the same skillet, dissolve another tablespoon of tallow. After that, brown ground chuck, crumbling with a spatula.

Include the vegetables back to the skillet; mix in the remaining ingredients. Set the heat to medium-low; simmer for 20 minutes; stirring every so often.

Enjoy over buns. Bon appétit!

Nutrition:

Calories: 313 Cal

Protein: 26.6 g

Fat: 20.6 g

Carbs: 3.5 g

Sugar: 0.3 g

Roasted Root Vegetables

Preparation Time: 10 minutes

Cooking Time: 1 hour and 30 minutes

Servings: 6

Ingredients:

2 tbsp. olive oil

1 head garlic, cloves separated and peeled

1 large turnip, peeled and cut into ½-inch pieces

1 medium-sized red onion, cut into ½-inch pieces

1 ½ lb. beets, trimmed but not peeled, scrubbed and cut into ½-inch pieces

1 ½ lb. Yukon gold potatoes, unpeeled, cut into ½-inch pieces

2 ½ lbs. butternut squash, peeled, seeded, cut into ½-inch pieces

Directions:

Grease 2 rimmed and large baking sheets. Preheat oven to 425oF.

In a huge bowl, mix all ingredients thoroughly.

Into the two baking sheets, evenly divide the root vegetables, spread in one layer.

Season generously with pepper and salt.

Place it into the oven, then roast for at least 1 hour and 15 minutes or until golden brown and tender.

Remove from the oven and let it cool for at least 15 minutes before serving.

Nutrition:

Calories 278

Total Fat 5g,
Saturated Fat 1g

Total Carbs 57g

Net Carbs 47g

Protein 6g

Sugar: 15g

Fiber 10g

Sodium 124mg

Potassium 1598mg

Stir-Fried Brussels Sprouts and Carrots

Preparation Time: 10 minutes
Cooking Time: 15 minutes
Servings: 6

Ingredients:

1 tbsp cider vinegar

1/3 cup water

1 lb. Brussels sprouts halved lengthwise

1 lb. carrots cut diagonally into ½-inch thick lengths

3 tbsp. olive oil, divided

2 tbsp. chopped shallot

½ tsp pepper ¾ tsp salt

Directions:

On medium-high fire, place a nonstick medium fry pan and heat 2 tbsp oil.

Ass shallots and cook until softened, around one to two minutes while occasionally stirring.

Add pepper salt, Brussels sprouts, and carrots. Stir fry until vegetables start to brown on the edges, around 3 to 4 minutes.

Add water, cook, and cover.

After 5 to 8 minutes, or when veggies are already soft, add remaining butter.

If needed, season with more pepper and salt to taste.

Turn off fire, transfer to a platter, serve and enjoy.

Nutrition:

Calories 98
Total Fat 4g
Saturated Fat 2g
Total Carbs 14g
Net Carbs 9g
Protein 3g
Sugar: 5g
Fiber 5g
Sodium 357mg

Potassium 502mg

Organic Asparagus Recipe

Preparation Time: 5 minutes

Cooking Time: 5 minutes

Servings: 2

Ingredients:

1 pound of asparagus

1 tbsp. buttered with grass (melted)

Unrefined sea salt

Pepper to taste

Directions:

Cut asparagus, this is easily accomplished by breaking off the ends where it naturally breaks off.

Pour the melted butter over asparagus and toss for coating.

Season generously with salt and pepper.

Place on a hot grill (medium heat) and grill for about 5-10 minutes until the asparagus is soft (turn frequently).

Nutrition:

Energy (calories): 63 kcal

Protein: 5.49 g

Fat: 1.02 g

Carbohydrates: 11.56 g

Zucchini Salad

Preparation Time: 25 minutes
Cooking Time: 0 minutes
Servings: 4

Ingredients:

2 zucchini

3 tablespoons mild olive oil

1 tbsp. balsamic vinegar

50 g of hazelnuts

15 g fresh basil

10 g of fresh mint

150 g burrata

Directions:

Cut the zucchini into 1 cm long slices. Season with salt and pepper and sprinkle with olive oil, heat the electric smoker and smoke the zucchini slices in 4 minutes. Turn halfway. Put the zucchini slices in a bowl, mix with the balsamic vinegar and let stand until use.

Heat a pan without oil or butter and roast the hazelnuts until golden brown for 3 minutes over medium heat. Cool on a plate and chop roughly.

Cut basil leaves and mint roughly. The stems of basil finely chop; they have a lot of taste. Mix the zucchini with the herbs and the rest of the oil. Tear the burrata to pieces.

Divide first the zucchini and then the burrata over the plates. Sprinkle with the roasted hazelnuts and herbs - season with (freshly ground) pepper and possibly salt.

Nutrition:

Energy (calories): 246 kcal

Protein: 2.93 g

Fat: 24.08 g

Carbohydrates: 6.7 g

Avocado Wrapped In Bacon

Preparation Time: 10 minutes
Cooking Time: 30 minutes
Servings: 4

Ingredients:

2 avocados (ripe)

15-20 strips of bacon

Directions:

For the avocado wrapped in bacon wrapped in bacon, first, Preheat your electric smoker to 225˚F.

Halve the avocado and remove the kernel. Carefully remove the pulp (preferably with a tablespoon). Then cut lengthwise into approximately 1 cm thick slits.

Wrap each column with a strip of bacon and place on the baking sheet. Put the avocado wrapped in bacon in the smoker until the bacon is crispy. Best observe because every oven is a little different.

Nutrition:

Energy (calories): 305 kcal

Protein: 5.8 g

Fat: 28.25 g

Carbohydrates: 13.27 g

Vegetable Skewers And Grilled Cheese

Preparation Time: 15 minutes

Cooking Time: 10 minutes

Servings: 4

Ingredients:

2 colored peppers, seeded and cut into cubes

340 g (3/4 lbs) Halloumi type grilled cheese, cubed

225 g (1/2 lb.) whole white mushrooms

30 ml (2 tablespoons) of olive oil

10 ml (2 teaspoons) balsamic vinegar

(1/2 teaspoon) of dried oregano

Directions:

Preheat the barbecue to medium-high power. Oil the grill.

In a bowl, mix all the ingredients. Salt and pepper.
Thread the vegetables alternately on skewers. Thread the cheese on other skewers. Reserve on a large plate.

Grill the vegetable for 10 minutes, turning them a few times during cooking with tongs. Oil the grate again. Grill the cheese skewers on both sides, turning them over as soon as the cheese begins to grill, about 1 minute on each side.

Serve immediately. Serve with pita bread, if desired.

Nutrition:

Energy (calories): 2063 kcal

Protein: 17.54 g

Fat: 220.73 g

Carbohydrates: 9.62 g

Seafood Salad And Salsa Verde With Thai Basil

Preparation Time: 25 minutes

Cooking Time: 8 minutes

Servings: 4

Ingredients:

- ✓ Salsa Verde
- ✓ 30 g (1 cup) Thai basil leaves
- ✓ 30 g (1 cup) coriander leaves
- ✓ 1/4 cup (60 mL) vegetable oil
- ✓ 45 ml (3 tablespoons) lime juice
- ✓ 30 ml (2 tablespoons) of water
- ✓ 1 green onion, cut into sections
- ✓ Seafood and vegetables
- ✓ 900 g (2 lbs) of mussels, cleaned
- ✓ 225 g (1/2 lbs) medium shrimp (31-40), shelled and deveined
- ✓ 4 small squid, trimmed
- ✓ 15 ml (1 tablespoon) vegetable oil
- ✓ 15 ml (1 tablespoon) lime juice
- ✓ 10 ml (2 teaspoons) fish sauce (nuoc-mam)
- ✓ 2 teaspoons (10 mL) turmeric
- ✓ 1 bulb of fennel, thinly sliced with mandolin
- ✓ 400 g (2 cups) baby potatoes, cooked
- ✓ 2 green onions, chopped
- ✓ 1 tomato, quartered
- ✓ Thai basil leaves, to taste

Directions:

Salsa Verde

In the electric smoker, finely grind all the ingredients.

Seafood and vegetables

Preheat the electric smoker to 225°F.

In a large bowl, combine mussels, shrimp, squid, oil, lime juice, fish sauce and turmeric. Salt and pepper.

Place the mussels directly on the electric smoker. Close it and cook the mussels until they are all open. Discard those that remain closed. Place in a bowl. Shell the mussels (keep some for service, if desired).

Grill shrimp and squid for 2 to 3 minutes per side or until shrimp and squid are cooked and browned. On a work surface, cut squid into 1 cm (1/2 inch) slices. Book.

Place the fennel in a bowl. Lightly oil, then season with salt and pepper.

Spread seafood and vegetables on plates. Sprinkle salsa Verde and garnish with Thai basil leaves.

Nutrition:

Energy (calories): 1456 kcal; Protein: 57.05 g;; Fat: 98.44 g; Carbohydrates: 112.61 g

BigGreenEgg - Stuffed Mussels On BBQ

Preparation Time: 10 minutes

Cooking Time: 20 minutes

Servings: 2

Ingredients:

- ✓ 2 kg of mussels
- ✓ 3/4 cup parmesan
- ✓ 1 C. ground pepper
- ✓ 1/2 cup of olive oil
- ✓ 1 cup of parsley
- ✓ 1 C. salt
- ✓ 6 cloves of garlic
- ✓ 1/2 nutmeg
- ✓ 1 cups of bread crumbs
- ✓ Sriracha sauce

Directions:

Step 1

Start the BBQ with indirect cooking (temperature about 400 F) cleaned the molds correctly.

(Remove the beard from the mussels) 2nd step

Place the mussels directly on the rack until it opens.

CAUTION: You must keep about 1/2 cup of the juice of your mussels.

When the mussels open, gently remove from the BBQ

Pour the sifted mold juice into a cup. measure.

Step 3

Remove all the mussels from their shells by keeping a half-shell as service plates.

Reserve the mussels and mix the rest of the ingredients together for your stuffing (Mold juice included) (without the mussels and without the sriracha)

Put a mussel in each shell and add your filling on top.

Nutrition:

Energy (calories): 3056 kcal

Protein: 268.92 g

Fat: 157.62 g

Carbohydrates: 129.1 g

Chapter 5: Snacks and Sides

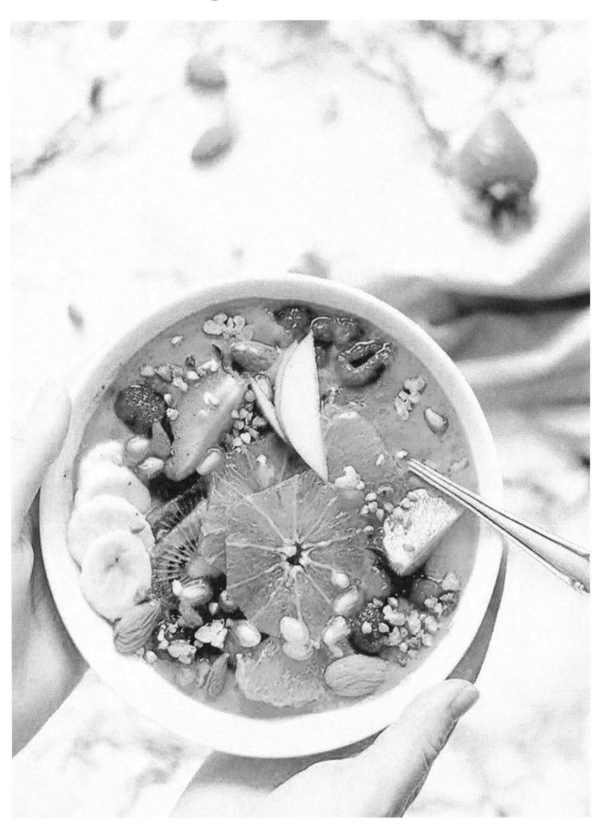

Low Cholesterol-Low Calorie Blueberry Muffin

Preparation Time: 10 minutes

Cooking Time: 25 minutes

Servings: 12

Ingredients:

1 cup blueberries, fresh

2 tablespoons melted margarine

2 teaspoons baking powder

1 and ½ cup of flour, all-purpose

1 egg white

½ cup skim milk or non-fat milk

1 tablespoon coconut oil

½ cup white sugar

Pinch of salt

Directions:

Set the oven to 205C.

Grease a 12-cup muffin pan using oil.

In a small bowl, place the blueberries. Add ¼ cup of the flour and mix it together. Set aside.

In another bowl, whisk the egg white and the coconut oil. Add the melted margarine.

In a separate bowl, mix all together the dry ingredients and sift. Sift again over the egg white mixture. Mix to moisten the flour. The flour should look lumpy, so do not overmix.

Fold in the blueberries. Separate the blueberries, so that each scoop will have blueberries. Scoop the mixture into the muffin pans. Fill only up to two-thirds of the pan.

Bake for 25 minutes or until the muffin turns golden brown.

Nutrition:

Calories: 114 kcal

Protein: 2.66 g

Fat: 5.34 g

Carbohydrates: 14.25 g

Carrot Sticks with Avocado Dip

Preparation Time: 10 minutes
Cooking Time: 0 minutes
Servings: 6

Ingredients:

1 large avocado, pitted

6 ounces shelled edamame

½ cup cilantro, tightly packed

½ onion

Juice of one lemon

2 tablespoon olive oil

1 tablespoon of chili-garlic sauce or chili sauce

Salt and pepper

Directions:

Place the edamame, cilantro, onion, and chili sauce in a blender or food processor. Pulse it to chop and mix the ingredients. Add the avocado and the lemon juice. Gradually add the olive oil as you blend. Transfer to a jar.

Scoop 2 spoons and serve with carrot sticks.

Nutrition:

Calories: 154 kcal

Protein: 5.16 g

Fat: 11.96 g

Carbohydrates: 8.44 g

Avocado-Apple-Prosciutto Wraps

Preparation Time: 15 minutes

Cooking Time: 0 minutes

Servings: 12

Ingredients:

✓ 12 slices prosciutto

✓ 2 large avocados, halved, pitted, and each half cut into 3 pieces

✓ 2 apples, each cut into 6 pieces (see Ingredient Tip)

✓ Raw honey, for drizzling (optional)

Directions:

Lay 1 slice of prosciutto on a plate with the short end closest to you. Place 1 avocado slice and 1 apple slice together at the short end of the prosciutto and roll it up, into a cigar shape. Repeat with the remaining ingredients.
Drizzle each wrap with honey (if using).

Nutrition:

Calories: 245;

Total Fat: 17g;

Saturated Fat: 4g;

Cholesterol: 50mg;

Garlicky Roasted Chickpeas

Preparation Time: 5 minutes

Cooking Time: 20 minutes

Servings: 4

Ingredients:

4 cups cooked (or canned) chickpeas, rinsed, drained, and thoroughly dried with paper towels (be careful not to crush them)

2 tablespoons extra-virgin olive oil

1 teaspoon salt

1 teaspoon garlic powder

Freshly ground black pepper

Directions:

Preheat the oven to 400°F.

Spread the chickpeas evenly on a rimmed baking sheet and coat them with the olive oil.

Bake for 20 minutes, stirring halfway through.

Transfer the hot chickpeas to a large bowl. Toss with the salt and garlic powder; season with pepper. Store leftovers in a sealed container or bag at room temperature; they'll remain crispy for 1 to 2 days.

Nutrition:

Calories: 150;

Total Fat: 5g;

Saturated Fat: 0g;

Cholesterol: 0mg;

<u>Creamy Polenta</u>

Preparation Time: 8 minutes

Cooking Time: 45 minutes

Servings: 4

Ingredients:

1 cup polenta

1 ½ cup water

2 cups chicken stock

½ cup cream

1/3 cup Parmesan, grated

Directions:

Put polenta in the pot.

Add water, chicken stock, cream, and Parmesan. Mix up polenta well.

Then preheat oven to 355F.

Cook polenta in the oven for 45 minutes.

Mix up the cooked meal with the help of the spoon carefully before serving.

Nutrition:

Calories 208

Fat 5.3

Fiber 1

Carbs 32.2

Protein 8

Mushroom Millet

Preparation Time: 10 minutes

Cooking Time: 15 minutes

Servings: 3

Ingredients:

¼ cup mushrooms, sliced ¾ cup onion, diced

1 tablespoon olive oil

1 teaspoon salt

3 tablespoons milk ½ cup millet

1 cup of water

1 teaspoon butter

Directions:

Pour olive oil in the skillet then put the onion.

Add mushrooms and roast the vegetables for 10 minutes over the medium heat. Stir them from time to time.

Meanwhile, pour water in the pan.

Add millet and salt.

Cook the millet with the closed lid for 15 minutes over the medium heat.

Then add the cooked mushroom mixture in the millet.

Add milk and butter. Mix up the millet well.

Nutrition:

Calories 198

Fat 7.7

Fiber 3.5

Carbs 27.9

Protein 4.7

Spicy Barley

Preparation Time: 7 minutes

Cooking Time: 42 minutes

Servings: 5

Ingredients:

1 cup barley

3 cups chicken stock

½ teaspoon cayenne pepper

1 teaspoon salt

½ teaspoon chili pepper

½ teaspoon ground black pepper

1 teaspoon butter

1 teaspoon olive oil

Directions:

Place barley and olive oil in the pan.

Roast barley on high heat for 1 minute. Stir it well.

Then add salt, chili pepper, ground black pepper, cayenne pepper, and butter. Add chicken stock.

Close the lid and cook barley for 40 minutes over the medium-low heat.

Nutrition:

Calories 152
Fat 2.9

Fiber 6.5

Carbs 27.8

Protein 5.1

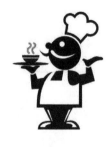

Tender Farro

Preparation Time: 8 minutes

Cooking Time: 40 minutes

Servings: 4

Ingredients:

1 cup farro

3 cups beef broth

1 teaspoon salt

1 tablespoon almond butter

1 tablespoon dried dill

Directions:

Place farro in the pan.

Add beef broth, dried dill, and salt.

Close the lid and place the mixture to boil.

Then boil it for 35 minutes over the medium-low heat.

When the time is done, open the lid and add almond butter.

Mix up the cooked farro well.

Nutrition:

Calories 95

Fat 3.3

Fiber 1.3

Carbs 10.1

Protein 6.4

Wheatberry Salad

Preparation Time: 10 minutes

Cooking Time: 50 minutes

Servings: 2

Ingredients:

¼ cup of wheat berries

1 cup of water

1 teaspoon salt

2 tablespoons walnuts, chopped

1 tablespoon chives, chopped

¼ cup fresh parsley, chopped

2 oz. pomegranate seeds

1 tablespoon canola oil

1 teaspoon chili flakes

Directions:

Place wheat berries and water in the pan.

Add salt and simmer the ingredients for 50 minutes over the medium heat.

Meanwhile, mix up together walnuts, chives, parsley, pomegranate seeds, and chili flakes. When the wheatberry is cooked, transfer it in the walnut mixture.

Add canola oil and mix up the salad well.

Nutrition:

Calories 160 Fat 11.8 Fiber 1.2 Carbs 12 Protein 3.4

Curry Wheatberry Rice

Preparation Time: 10 minutes

Cooking Time: 1 hour 15 minutes

Servings: 5

Ingredients:

1 tablespoon curry paste

¼ cup milk

1 cup wheat berries

½ cup of rice

1 teaspoon salt

4 tablespoons olive oil

6 cups chicken stock

Directions:

Place wheatberries and chicken stock in the pan.

Close the lid and cook the mixture for 1 hour over the medium heat.

Then add rice, olive oil, and salt.

Stir well.

Mix up together milk and curry paste.

Add the curry liquid in the rice-wheatberry mixture and stir well.

Boil the meal for 15 minutes with the closed lid.

When the rice is cooked, all the meal is cooked.

Nutrition:

Calories 232

Fat 15

Fiber 1.4

Carbs 23.5

Protein 3.9

Day	Breakfast	Lunch	Dinner
1	Cranberry and Raisins Granola	Rosemary Chicken Thighs	Eggplant Cannelloni
2	Tomato Bruschetta with Basil	Tomato & Cheese Chicken Chili	Spicy Habanero and Ground Beef Dinner
3	Mango Granola	Salmon and Scallions	Grilled Beef Angus And Chorizo
4	Bake Apple Turnover	Greek Prosciutto-Wrapped Meatloaf	Oregano Pork
5	Tomato and Avocado Omelet	Chicken and Mushroom Salad	Organic Asparagus Recipe
6	Vegan-Friendly Banana Bread	Flying Jacob Casserole	Meatballs with Roasted Peppers and Manchego
7	Spicy Marble Eggs	Feta & Bacon Chicken	Parsley Pork and Artichokes
8	Apple Bruschetta with Almonds and Blackberries	Cod and Peas	The Best Sloppy Joes Ever
9	Quinoa and Cauliflower Congee	Chili Snapper	Roasted Root Vegetables
10	Buckwheat Pancakes with Vanilla Almond Milk	Salmon and Carrots	Seafood Salad And Salsa Verde With Thai Basil
11	Brown Sugar Cinnamon Oatmeal	BBQ Chicken Zucchini Boats	Vegetable Skewers And Grilled Cheese

12	Beef Breakfast Casserole	Greek-Style Cold Beef Salad	Stir-Fried Brussels Sprouts and Carrots
13	Nutty Oats Pudding	Lemony Mackerel	Spicy Habanero and Ground Beef Dinner
14	Oven-Poached Eggs	Turkey Stew	BigGreenEgg - Stuffed Mussels On BBQ
15	Buckwheat Pancakes with Vanilla Almond Milk	Chili Snapper	Organic Asparagus Recipe
16	Vegan-Friendly Banana Bread	Feta & Bacon Chicken	Roasted Root Vegetables
17	Tomato and Avocado Omelet	Greek-Style Cold Beef Salad	Eggplant Cannelloni
18	Quinoa and Cauliflower Congee	Chicken and Mushroom Salad	Oregano Pork
19	Apple Bruschetta with Almonds and Blackberries	Lemony Mackerel	Vegetable Skewers And Grilled Cheese
20	Cranberry and Raisins Granola	Salmon and Carrots	Spicy Habanero and Ground Beef Dinner
21	Nutty Oats Pudding	BBQ Chicken Zucchini Boats	Parsley Pork and Artichokes
22	Bake Apple Turnover	Salmon and Scallions	Spicy Habanero and Ground Beef Dinner
23	Oven-Poached Eggs	Cod and Peas	Seafood Salad And Salsa Verde With Thai Basil

24	Spicy Marble Eggs	Turkey Stew	BigGreenEgg - Stuffed Mussels On BBQ
25	Beef Breakfast Casserole	Rosemary Chicken Thighs	Grilled Beef Angus And Chorizo
26	Tomato Bruschetta with Basil	Tomato & Cheese Chicken Chili	Meatballs with Roasted Peppers and Manchego
27	Mango Granola	Flying Jacob Casserole	Stir-Fried Brussels Sprouts and Carrots
8	Brown Sugar Cinnamon Oatmeal	Greek Prosciutto-Wrapped Meatloaf	The Best Sloppy Joes Ever

Conclusion

Thank you for making it through to the end of the Anti-Inflammatory Diet Cookbook. Let's hope it was informative and able to provide you with all of the tools you must attain your goals, whatever they may be. Inflammation is a normal process of our immune system and completely necessary to protect us from threats that will damage our cells and tissues. If it weren't for our immune system, our bodies would be ravaged instantly by deadly diseases, and the results would be fatal. As long as the inflammatory process does not last beyond its normal time, there is usually no issue. Once the inflammation becomes chronic or long-term, it becomes an inflammatory disease and will create damaging results.

The inflammatory disease will lead to many different health consequences and will even attack our most vital organs. The best way to do this is to prevent chronic inflammation in the first place. The next best thing is to recognize the signs and symptoms as early as possible, so proper interventions can be done to limit and reverse the impact of chronic inflammation. Inflammatory disease is the root cause of many long-term diseases, so ignoring the warning signs can create major consequences for your health.

Unfortunately, if the inflammatory disease gets out of control, preventative measures may be out of the question, and medical interventions will need to be done. Our goal is to prevent you from getting to this point. Lucky for us, many lifestyle changes can be performed to stop and reverse this disease process when it is still in its in advance stages. This is another reason why we should recognize and not ignore the signs and symptoms. A major lifestyle change we can commit to is a new diet plan. The anti-inflammatory diet is a meal plan that boasts healthy and nutritious cuisines, but still flavorful and appealing to the taste buds. There is a major myth out there that healthy food cannot be delicious. We have proven this myth wrong by providing numerous recipes from around the world that follow our healthy meal plan.

We hope that the information you read in this book gives you a better understanding of how the immune system functions and how a proper diet plan can help protect it and our other valuable cells and tissues. The recipes we have provided are just a starting point. Use them as a guide to create many of your dishes that follow the diet plan. Just make sure you use the proper ingredients and food groups. Also, for maximum results, follow the Anti-Inflammatory Diet food guide.

The next step is to take the instruction we have provided and begin taking steps to change your life and improve your health. Begin recognizing the signs and symptoms of chronic inflammation and make the necessary lifestyle changes to prevent further health problems. Start transitioning to the anti-inflammatory diet today by incorporating small meals into your schedule and increase the amount as tolerated. Within a short period, the diet will be a regular part of your routine. You will notice increased energy, improved mental function, a stronger and well-balanced immune system, reduction in chronic pain, some healthy weight loss, and overall better health outcomes. If you are ready to experience these changes, then wait no longer and begin putting your knowledge from this book into action.

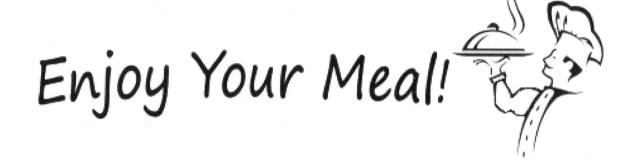

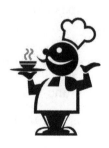